THE
MENOPAUSE
COMPANION

THE MENOPAUSE COMPANION

A BEGINNER'S GUIDE TO OWNING YOUR TRANSITION, FROM PERI TO POST

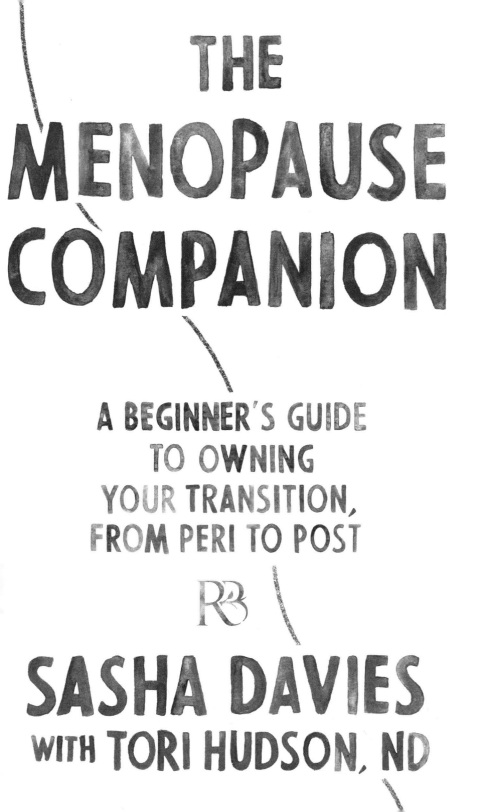

RB

SASHA DAVIES

WITH TORI HUDSON, ND

Roost Books
An imprint of Shambhala Publications, Inc.
2129 13th Street
Boulder, Colorado 80302
www.roostbooks.com

Note: The information presented in this book is for educational purposes only
and is not intended to diagnose or treat any health conditions. Please consult
your health practitioner regarding any specific health concerns and care.

Cover art: Nina Simoneaux
Cover design: Nina Simoneaux
Interior design: Amy Sly

9 8 7 6 5 4 3 2 1

First Edition
Printed in Malaysia

Shambhala Publications makes every effort to print on acid-free, recycled paper.
Roost Books is distributed worldwide by Penguin Random House, Inc., and
its subsidiaries.

Library of Congress Cataloging-in-Publication Data

Names: Davies, Sasha, author. | Hudson, Tori, author.
Title: The menopause companion: a beginner's guide to owning your
    transition, from peri to post / Sasha Davies with Tori Hudson, ND.
Description: First edition. | Boulder, Colorado: Roost Books, an imprint
    of Shambhala Publications, Inc., [2023] | Includes bibliographical
    references.
Identifiers: LCCN 2022025982 | ISBN 9781611809831 (trade paperback)
Subjects: LCSH: Menopause—Popular works.
Classification: LCC RG186 .D358 2023 | DDC 618.1/75—dc23/eng/20220713
LC record available at https://lccn.loc.gov/2022025982

CONTENTS

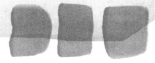

PREFACE

What do you do when someone you have never met asks you to participate in what sounds like a big project: co-writing a book? You have a full work schedule and then some, you are raising a child, and . . . it's COVID times. You just say *no*. But then I spoke on the phone with Sasha Davies, and though every fiber in my being wanted to say no, some different fiber grew during our chat. I said yes.

In that first conversation, it was clear that what Sasha wanted to bring forth in this book was unique. It wasn't just menopause physiology, symptoms, and treatment options with a list of dos and don'ts or better this and not that. In addition to the more medical side of things, Sasha wanted to emphasize how perimenopause and menopause are *actually* experienced.

That outlook plus my near forty years of experience in natural medicine, integrative medicine, and women's health and expertise, specifically in menopause and menopausal hormonal therapy, made me a natural fit to assist Sasha in writing this book.

Though it's difficult to pinpoint a specific moment when I decided to focus on menopause care within the field of women's health, it's easy to see how the dots connect when I look back at my journey. Ever since I began menstruating—at 2 p.m. on November 24, 1964, when I was twelve years old—I have been waiting for menopause! I noticed early in my career that women going through the transition to menopause were not being adequately helped by their OB/GYNs, who are most adept at reproductive-age issues, nor by family practice doctors and internists, who have plenty of other health issues to manage in their patients. Nor was the alternative medicine community very sophisticated in offering consistently effective herbal or nutritional solutions. In addition, menopause-related hormone therapy research and prescribing were going through big shifts that were opening up questions about safety and efficacy. No matter who the practitioner was, we were all limited by the lack of research on midlife women. This was in the mid-1980s, before Congress passed legislation mandating that the National Institutes of Health (NIH) ensure women and minorities be included in government-funded research and permanently established the NIH Office of Research on Women's Health (ORWH).

I was highly motivated to help the women who were seeking answers to alleviate their suffering, and I made menopause a specialty in my clinical practice, professional education, mentoring, writing, and research. As scientific evidence for natural therapies began to emerge in the late 1980s and research in menopause hormone management evolved in significant ways, I found more and more high-quality answers and solutions to help my patients. I found this immensely satisfying. It was my patients who led me on this path of integrating natural and conventional therapies, weighing the benefits and risks of each, and seeing how they are best combined for what each individual needs.

At my clinic in Portland, Oregon, called A Woman's Time, I have helped tens of thousands of women over the years. As an adjunct clinical professor at four different medical schools of naturopathic medicine, I have educated thousands of licensed naturopathic physicians. Through my research endeavors, publications and lectures, and clinical practice, I have felt privileged—again, thanks to my patients—to become an expert on perimenopause and menopause evaluation and management using botanicals, nutraceuticals, and hormonal medication options. I have also made it part of my career to work with, learn from, and lecture to conventional medical doctors, taking a leadership role in integrating conventional and natural medicine through the National Institutes of Health and other integrative medicine training programs. I have a passion and drive to foster conversation and learning, with a view of advancing the field of women's health.

This book is the product of Sasha's robust, diligent, and persistent research and collaboration: she consulted books, articles, and scientific publications; spoke directly with women in about their experiences; and engaged in frequent and extended conversations with me. One of the many things I appreciated about working with Sasha was her ability to ask questions in a way that helped me see gaps and explain things better. It was a learning experience for both of us! Sasha is insightful and articulate in interpreting scientific information into an easy-to-understand format and making complex ideas both very accessible and personally relevant. She has been able to interpret the multitude of experiences of perimenopause and menopause as more than just physiology by reflecting the personal journey that these experiences create—both the good and the bad.

We collaborated on this project during the pandemic. I think we met in person only once, but that didn't stop a fruitful relationship from blossoming into this book. After many hours of conversations and scores of emails back and forth, it is something I feel extremely fortunate to have been a part of. This book does indeed offer something new in the terrain of perimenopause and menopause, with a fresh view on both medical and real-life experiences of it as well as guidance to facilitate decision-making. Sasha's ability to write with clarity, freshness, sensitivity, transparency, cleverness, and humor truly delights and inspires me.

Whether you are reading this before the onset of perimenopause, throughout perimenopause, or postmenopause, this book will serve as a guide and companion. It doesn't offer a specific road map for the best path through the menopause process—as you'll see, menopause is such an individualized experience that such a map cannot exist. Rather this book will support you in tuning in to your body, collecting data, sharing information with clinicians, and using what you learn to make decisions you can feel good about. After all, as Sasha says, it's not your mom's menopause, your friend's menopause, or your doctor's menopause. It's yours. This guide provides guidance and companionship for your unique journey.

Prepare to learn, feel supported, and become empowered.

Tori Hudson, ND
Clinical professor at National University of Natural Medicine, Bastyr University, Canadian College of Naturopathic Medicine, and Southwest College of Naturopathic Medicine
Author of *Women's Encyclopedia of Natural Medicine*
Medical director at A Woman's Time clinic
www.drtorihudson.com

INTRODUCTION

Menopause has been rebranded numerous times over the course of history—as a condition of toxicity resulting from menstrual blood retention, as the tragic end of femininity, as an opportunity to reinvent oneself—and thus each generation relates to it slightly differently. Even with all these fluctuations, one characteristic of the experience remains stubbornly the same: menopause seems mysterious. Generation after generation have wondered in whispers and shouts, *What is this thing, and why isn't anyone talking about it?*

As someone who has spent the past few years surveying the landscape of menopause information, I can say with confidence that we know what it is (though not everything about how it affects the body) and people are talking about it. Kind of a lot, actually. Books, magazines, patient brochures, and product companies are offering overviews of physiology, potential symptoms, and treatment options, and although this content seems like exactly what's needed to demystify menopause, it leaves a lot to be desired.

When you ask what menopause will be like, what you're really asking is a similar but distinct question: *What will menopause be like for me?* Your question cannot be fully answered with the generalized information we have about physiology, symptoms, and treatments because any satisfactory reply, in addition to predicting *your* body's precise response to menopause (which isn't possible), must also address the other forces at play in menopause, the ones outside the borders of your flesh and bones and inside our culture and institutions. The uncertainty surrounding menopause is not only about what will happen within your body but also the interaction between your body and the perceptions and demands of the world.

It's difficult to fully grasp how it feels when a place that is intimately familiar to you—your body, including its routines and your sense of self—changes in ways that are beyond your control. The transition to menopause is not a virus or a disease. It's a complex physiological process that, like both of those things, impacts the

individual lives it touches in dramatically different ways. That idiosyncrasy makes it challenging to prepare yourself, because you don't know exactly what's coming. Will you have hot flashes or insomnia? Will you be liberated from your concerns about what other people think? Will your vulva still get wet when you're turned on—wait, will you even *want* sex anymore?

Medical professionals will tell you not to fret, it's a natural and normal transition, but articles you read and people you talk to about their experiences of menopause tell a murkier story. All of them are telling the truth. Menopause can be a powerful experience whether it's mystical and magical, rough going, or a bit of both. Your experience of it isn't the result of any one thing you've done or an inner strength you possess, and it's as much about the hand you were dealt—including genetics, class, culture, and geography—as how you played it. No one can predict how your transition to menopause will unfold, and if someone tells you they can, I encourage you to politely say *no thank you* to whatever they're selling.

I've been carefully observing menopause since I watched two good friends get shaken up by their transitions a few years ago. As I listened to them describe their struggles with physical symptoms that disrupted their daily lives, it dawned on me that I knew next to nothing about this transition that I too would go through someday. Finding basics in books and on the internet was easy: end of ovulation, end of periods, end of fertility. There were lists of potential symptoms and familiar platitudes about taking good care of oneself. All of it came across like a pamphlet your doctor might hand you on your way out of their office—basic and overgeneralized to the point of *why bother*. When I held that up against the experiences of the women I knew who were going through it, there was a disconnect.

Although I hadn't experienced the physical tumult of night sweats, insomnia, or hormonal migraines that my friends were reporting, there was something intimately familiar about the tenor of their experience. It looked a lot like the distress I have felt in the face of big life changes—a move, a new or lost job, a breakup—the kind that upend my sense of stability and force me to reconsider who I am.

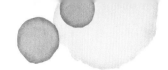

My friends were fighting to be seen and heard by their partners and practitioners alike, but their outrage was wobbly with the kind of self-doubt that lurks around the edges of new and unfamiliar experiences. They seemed unsure of whether their feelings were reasonable or a bit too much. This aspect of the menopause transition is decidedly less visible in pamphlet-land, even though it appeared to be the backdrop for my friends' entire experience.

Menopause is a physiological transition that unfolds in our bodies—often during midlife but sometimes earlier—with real physical changes and symptoms that can be disruptive to aspects of daily life including sleep, cognition, and comfort. And modern menopause is also a social construct interwoven with narratives about femininity that are rooted in patriarchal and white supremacist ideologies and that operate within a capitalist system. Every change that menopause brings, big or small, is lived out in the life of a person in a body with intersecting identities, a unique reproductive history, and an understanding of themselves in relationship to the world. All these tendrils are tangled up and inseparable, and thus the experience of menopause is different across cultures and also within a culture depending on the body it's happening in: queer, white, with a disability, Black, skinny, Asian, and so on.

Once I saw that menopause is a transition in a person's life rather than something confined to their physiology, the most pressing question became: what would someone going through it need—in addition to an understanding of their body—to feel prepared? This is not a question with a singular answer; rather, it's a territory to be mapped. That's what I've attempted to do in this guide: to make the landscape of menopause, including and beyond the physiology, more visible.

If you are reading this before or at the onset of menopause, think of this guide as a supportive companion for your journey, not a map of the right, best, or easiest path through menopause. Although I can't tell you how your menopause experience will go, I will provide information and tools to support you in listening to yourself—your body and your thoughts—so that you can employ that expertise in making decisions along the way. I want you to feel prepared to have *your* menopause, not the one your best friend is having, the one your mom had, the one you read about in a magazine, or the one the doctor described.

Our perceptions and experiences of menopause are bound up with cultural expectations and beliefs about female bodies, femininity, race, class, and the principles of capitalism, including productivity, power, and profit. It's a difficult web to untangle, as all these things are at play in our understanding of the transition to menopause. I have focused on the aspects of menopause that American culture has the most entrenched beliefs about or resistance toward because they are the primary ideas feeding our fears about menopause and aging. If you do not see your specific experience reflected here, that does not mean it's less valid or challenging, only that it occupies a less visible part of the territory.

I used to struggle to describe the impacts of menopause to people who have not experienced it. Now I simply begin by asking if they remember the onset of the COVID-19 pandemic: a constellation of uninvited and often difficult changes that arrived without an expiration date, making it hard to ignore and even harder to know how much time and attention to invest in accommodating it. I ask them to recall how everyone, for a variety of reasons, experienced it differently, from variations of grief and sadness to glimpses of new possibilities from the depths of all that change.

Then I say, yeah, menopause is kind of like that.

Though there is uncertainty on the path ahead, there are also ways you can prepare yourself. Knowledge of how the body works and the options for getting relief will help, and that's all here within this guide. But, as we've seen through the pandemic, in order to process what we experience, we need and want more than an understanding of biological basics and directives to be careful. That's why this guide also focuses on helping you develop an understanding of *your* body, your individual context for menopause, and how to build the kind of internal and external support systems you're likely to need (plus the confidence required to call on them when needed). If there is anything the pandemic can offer to our larger understanding of menopause, it's that comfort and support are not only meaningful but essential in times of transition. In other words, when you can't know how it's going to go, it helps to know and trust what you can lean into.

You don't always have control over when and how menopause transpires in your body, and that can be frustrating. It's hard to embrace a journey (even one that's natural and normal) that you didn't choose for yourself. There are many ways to set yourself up for an easier go of things, and we will explore those together at length. Although I can't answer the existential question of *Why me?*, I can address that question literally by explaining our current understanding of what the body does on the path to menopause and why. In fact, that's where we'll begin.

In part one we will examine the physiology of the ovaries and uterus over the course of one's lifetime and some of the external forces, such as culture and capitalism, that set the tone and context for the menopause transition. This foundation of information prepares us to explore what the experience of menopause can look like in an individual body and life, which we will do in part two. Finally, in part three we will discuss ways of tending to physical, logistical, and emotional needs.

Before we dive in, I want to acknowledge that taking care of your body is not a game played on a level field. We don't all have access to the same choices, in the care we solicit or the care we are able to give to ourselves, and even if we do have access, we don't all receive the same quality of treatment or get the help we need to apply generalized information to our unique situation. Every intervention discussed in this guide requires resources. Even things that seem universally accessible, like growing an awareness of what's happening in your body or reaching out to people in your network for help, are more or less so depending on your circumstances.

Throughout the guide, we are going to prod and examine how the experience of menopause is shaped and reshaped by the relationship between your body and the world around you. This exploration is messy because the boundaries of the menopause experience are blurred, making it difficult to pinpoint precise causes and effects. As you move through the information, I encourage you to hold this question in your mind: what would be possible if we presumed that the body going through menopause is not the problem, but the absence of adequate support for and unrealistic expectations of that body are what make the volatility of the menopause transition untenable?

The unknowns of your menopause will not be revealed until you experience them, but hopefully by making the forces that shape them more visible we can render them less mysterious, or at the very least we can begin to imagine a society and a world that could (and would) better accommodate the mystery.

AUTHOR'S NOTE

Throughout the process of writing this guide, I had the good fortune to partner with Dr. Tori Hudson, ND, a naturopathic practitioner specializing in women's health. I believe that the combination of my perspective as a layperson navigating the menopause landscape and her decades of experience as a clinician and educator made it possible to fully explore the lived experience of menopause. In addition to extensive conversations with Dr. Hudson, I conducted formal interviews with a dozen individuals and spoke informally with dozens more.

I decided not to ask my interviewees for any identifying information—not gender, sexuality, disability, socioeconomic standing, age, or race. I did learn some of that information about a few individuals from details they made explicit during our conversations. This is how I know that I spoke with white, Black, Asian, cisgender, heterosexual, and queer people about their menopause experiences. While I did first sit with the question of what you, the reader, might gain by having all that identifying information, I did not arrive at a clear reason to ask for it. As much as every aspect of a person's identity informs their menopause experience, it does not determine it for that individual or for others with similar identities; this made me hesitant to explicitly connect the experiences of individuals with the components of their identity. In some ways,

I thought, it could reveal a relatedness, but it also seemed to have as much potential to alienate or to set false expectations of similar experiences.

I am not a sociologist or a formally trained qualitative researcher, and the excerpts of these interviews do not (and are not intended to) account for all possible experiences in menopause. That's not intended as an excuse; it's a reality that would be true even with a group of interviewees ten times the size. I chose to weave their voices into the text because the voices of those who go through menopause are notably absent from so much of the literature surrounding the topic. The goal of sharing pieces of these conversations is to give texture and an expanded vocabulary to an experience often described by medical professionals in clinical terms.

My interview questions were inspired by the pioneering work of Kristen M. Swanson, RN, PhD, who began conducting research in the 1980s that brought the lived experience of miscarriage into the awareness of clinicians and the public. Each interviewee responded to a pair of prompts—"What's it like?" "What made you feel cared for?"—in the way that made sense to them. The words of the individuals who shared their experiences with me are highlighted throughout the book; I changed their names but none of their words.

The information I've shared about the physiological process of menopause and its accompanying symptoms is based on science and research that does not delineate between cisgender, transgender, and nonbinary experiences. Note that all my interviewees referred to themselves as women; as such, I use "women" and "she" throughout this text while understanding that not everyone who experiences menopause identifies as a woman, and not all women—including transgender women—will experience menopause in the same way.

PART ONE

|

What Is Menopause?

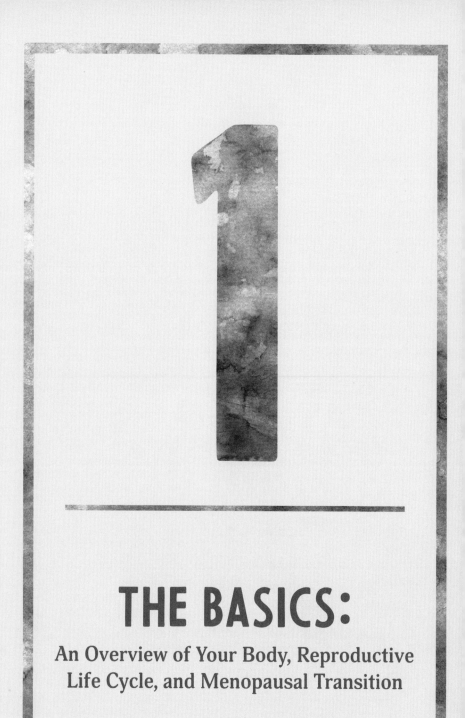

1

THE BASICS:

An Overview of Your Body, Reproductive
Life Cycle, and Menopausal Transition

Menopause is the official marker of the end of your fertility. I think of it as puberty's rowdy older sister. The term *menopause* refers to the one-year anniversary of your final menstrual period. *Perimenopause* is the transition process that leads up to the official marker of menopause. It begins around the time you start noticing a variety of changes in your body, and it can last up to a decade. During perimenopause, your body is working to adapt to changes in your sex hormone levels. There is some confusion about these terms though, because *menopause* is also often used as an umbrella term that encompasses both of these things.

Some doctors call perimenopause *second puberty*. The association makes sense considering that both are transitions driven by a shift in sex hormone levels that reverberates through the entire body, creating physiological changes that may inspire new or strong feelings about ourselves and our relationship to the world around us. As you will see, your sex hormones are powerful substances with huge influence throughout your body. It takes time and energy for your whole body to recalibrate itself when your hormone levels change.

"I didn't realize I wasn't a teenager until my teenage stepdaughter started living with us, and I was like, *Oh, I am not a teenager anymore.* And that was probably right when perimenopause was starting. I felt like I could see the reflection of what was happening in her." —SHEILA

MENOPAUSE TYPES

People who have heard scary stories of challenging symptoms and struggles sometimes want to know if they can skip menopause. Nearly all people with female anatomy will experience menopause, but they will all experience it differently. Overall health (including any medical conditions and treatments), life experiences, genetics, and environment are all factors in determining the nature, intensity, duration, and meaning of this transition. Although it is impossible to predict the details of any one path to menopause, we do know that all experiences fall into one of these types.

NATURAL

If you begin perimenopause after age forty-five without any medical intervention, once you haven't had a period for one full year, you will have experienced natural menopause. "Natural" does not mean better, normal, gradual, without treatment, or that the one-year anniversary of your last period will happen at fifty-one, the current average age. The word *natural* only means that your body initiated and completed this process within the age range medical professionals expect based on data collected through research.

The transition to menopause can last anywhere from two to ten years. Each transition is unique and dynamic; symptoms can come and go, and their intensity can increase or decrease over time. Most, but not all, people experience a tapering off of perimenopause symptoms such as mood swings, brain fog, and hot flashes in the first couple years following their final menstrual period.

INDUCED OR MEDICAL

You can also enter menopause as the result of a surgical removal of both ovaries (bilateral oophorectomy), a treatment for disease like pelvic radiation or chemotherapy, or hormone-blocking medications for cancer or pelvic disorders. In this scenario there is less or possibly no transition period for the body because ovarian function comes to a sudden halt. Such a dramatic shift can intensify symptoms. Because the changes that accompany menopause are caused by shifts in hormone levels, not age, medical menopause can happen at any age beyond puberty. In fact, removal of your uterus (hysterectomy) or even just one of your ovaries can make menopause begin earlier.

Menopause can also be induced via pharmacological intervention like gender-affirming hormone therapy (HT). Transgender women or nonbinary people using estrogens as HRT could experience symptoms similar to those of people in menopause if their hormone therapy, designed to increase estrogen, is interrupted. Transgender men or nonbinary people using testosterone as HRT will also go through a cessation of menses akin to menopause. How these experiences relate to cisgender women's menopausal transitions are not well studied yet, although hopefully one day we will all learn from each other's journeys through hormonal and physiological change.

PREMATURE

If the one-year anniversary of your last menstrual period is before the age of forty, you will probably hear the phrase "premature ovarian insufficiency" (POI). There are multiple potential causes for menstrual periods to stop, one of which is consistently elevated levels of follicle-stimulating hormone (FSH)—an indicator of the arrival of menopause. A diagnosis of premature menopause requires that your practitioner follow a protocol (a clinical workup) to rule out other potential causes. For example, menstruation can stop because of a thyroid disorder or another autoimmune condition, a prolactin-secreting tumor, nutrient deficiency and weight loss resulting from excessive physical exercise, disordered eating, or excessive stress. Note that genetics plays a role here too; some bodies are genetically predisposed to enter menopause at an earlier age than others.

Menstruation is an indicator of reproductive function and hormonal activity that impacts other systems within your body. If menstruation stops earlier than anticipated, it's important to get to the root cause of that significant change in the body, whether that is indeed premature menopause or something else.

"I think the experience for me has been a little bit shocking and jarring. This started coming up when I was forty, and I wasn't expecting to start having major night sweats every night. I didn't expect to be told by doctors that I was no longer fertile. I didn't really know that would impact me the way that it did, but it really impacts your identity as a woman—I would never have known that. I still sort of thought of myself being young. I was maybe more prepared for a transition like this to happen later."

—KRISTIN

EARLY

If the one-year anniversary of your final menstrual cycle happens between ages forty and forty-five, your menopause is considered early. Early menopause is often the result of induced or medical menopause; however, 3 to 5 percent of the population will arrive at menopause early without medical or pharmacological intervention.

Note that, if you skip more than two consecutive periods and you are not pregnant, it doesn't mean you are in early menopause (or that you have a disease). However, it can be a signal from your body that something needs attention, so it's a good idea to see a medical professional. Stress, hypo- or hyperthyroidism, malnutrition, pituitary disease, and polycystic ovarian disease are some of the other nonmenopausal causes of missed periods.

A NOTE ABOUT "EVERY" BODY

The concept of "normal" or "average" in medicine is a relatively new one. As Sara Hendren shares in her book *What Can a Body Do? How We Meet the Built World*, before the nineteenth century we compared all bodies to the unattainable physique and strength of gods, goddesses, and heroes. When statistical averaging tools used in astronomy were applied to humans by French statistician Adolphe Quetelet, it ultimately led to the practice of comparing human bodies to one another. Hendren acknowledges the power of statistics to help us ferret out and predict patterns—traffic, weather, infectious disease—but notes that "the habit of statistical thinking, broadly applied, creates a distancing effect, obscuring the specificities that also matter." Averages can lead researchers, and us, to presume much more sameness amid a group than is true. She sums it up nicely: "While facts that mark a group are valuable, statistics tell us nothing about the lives of individual people."

Our bodies are similar in so many ways, and that has allowed us to learn a lot about human physiology—the mechanics of how our bodies do all that they do. For example, all bodies are made up of cells, they need oxygen and water, they've got veins with blood pumping through them, and so on. But there are also differences between bodies, and those differences are incredibly important. Even one difference can mean a dramatically different lived experience: skin color, an XX or XY chromosome combo, height, blood that doesn't clot, a peanut allergy. As a result, there is no one-size-fits-all guide to the human body, which makes learning about *the body* and understanding *your body* very different endeavors.

The reality is that our experiences of bodily functions and physiological changes are distributed across a broad spectrum. Each summary that highlights one small area where the most dots are clustered together perpetuates the notion of a normal or average experience. It's understandable to start by discussing the clusters, but when the conversation stops there, it can make people who have a different experience feel like something is wrong with them. We're going to talk about differences a lot here.

MENOPAUSE HIGHLIGHTS

1. THE END OF FERTILITY

If puberty is the on-ramp to your fertile years, when you have periods and can make babies, then menopause is the corresponding off-ramp. At some point in midlife, your ovaries begin to slow down and eventually stop maturing and releasing eggs. (Remember, this can also happen suddenly as a result of a medical intervention.) When there are no eggs, there can be no babies. Researchers are not certain why we go through menopause (though there are theories), but they do know that the activity at the center of it—the main event—is the aging of the ovaries.

2. NO MORE PERIODS

When your ovaries retire, the ongoing hormonal dance they've been in with your brain (specifically the hypothalamus) and an aspect of your endocrine system (the pituitary gland) grinds to a halt. Without that dance, sex hormones are not directing the cells lining your uterus to build a warm and welcoming wall and then to shed it when no egg shows up.

3. YOU MIGHT HAVE SOME SYMPTOMS

Changes in the activities of your ovaries affect the production and distribution of important hormones—estrogen, progesterone, and testosterone—that manage processes in your reproductive system *and* throughout the rest of your body. The menopause transition often happens midlife, when we first begin to see signs of age-related changes, some of which are exacerbated by the hormonal fluctuations of menopause. The most common symptoms reported in the U.S. by people entering the menopause transition are:

Hot flashes and night sweats: Both of these are disruptions to the thermostat that regulates your body temperature, leading to overheating and chilling.

Vaginal dryness: Changes to the cells in the vagina can cause itching and burning sensations or make penetration painful.

Changes in body shape and size: During the menopausal transition, there is a tendency for fat to accumulate around the midsection, just above the pelvic area. Lean muscle mass also declines, which makes it even easier for fat to accumulate in the body.

4. IT'S BASICALLY A GIANT RECALIBRATION

Our bodies can adapt to new conditions—both internal and external—but it doesn't happen overnight. Imagine you are right-handed and are suddenly forced to switch to doing everything with your left hand. It's possible, but not without time and some fumbling along the way. Cells all over your body are accustomed to receiving specific levels of estrogen and progesterone at regular intervals throughout your menstrual cycle. So, they can react in a variety of ways to the hormonal peaks and valleys of the transition before eventually stabilizing around lower hormone levels.

5. THOUGH THERE ARE SYMPTOMS, IT'S NOT A DISEASE

The medical definition of *disease* is murky, but our cultural understanding is clear: disease means that someone is sick, and being sick means that something is happening in your body that's not supposed to happen. Menopause is a process that our bodies are designed to go through. Although the menopausal transition can include symptoms that make you feel unwell—lack of sleep, anxiety, joint pain—that does not make menopause a disease. There is a big gap between sick and thriving: if you are experiencing symptoms that are disrupting your life, your practitioner should work with you to identify the root causes and support you in implementing strategies to mitigate those symptoms.

YOUR EQUIPMENT

Every living being has a life span beginning with birth, ending with death, and riddled with activity in between. Most living things reproduce until they die. Humans don't; we evolved to outlive our reproductive capabilities. Menstrual cycles are part of a larger arc (the life cycle) of the reproductive system that includes multiple stages, each with a unique set of activities. Fertility—ovulation and menstruation—is something we have access to only for part of our lives; our reproductive system transitions from infertility to fertility (via puberty) and back again (via perimenopause) over the course of our lifetime.

Before we get into how to navigate potential symptoms and experiences associated with the transition to menopause, let's review reproductive anatomy and each phase of the life cycle of the reproductive system. Understanding how this system functions and interacts with the rest of the body will lay the groundwork for making sense of the impacts you might experience when those functions change.

You've probably seen cross-sections of the internal and external female sex organs in textbooks, an encyclopedia, or the posters hanging on the exam room walls at your doctor's office. The frontal view loosely resembles a steer's skull, and the view from the side looks something like a misshapen bag with a few folded gummy worms inside. Let's go over the names and functions of each part and describe the area of the body they inhabit in a bit more detail.

VULVA

The vulva includes so much more than it gets credit for: the mons pubis, the mound over your pubic bone that develops hair during puberty; the labia majora and labia minora, two sets of lips or folds in the skin that protect the openings of the urethra and the vagina; the clitoris, a mass of enervated tissue; and the perineum, a small patch of flesh between the base of the lips and the anus. The area beneath the inner labia minora, with openings to the vagina and the urethra, is called the vestibule.

VAGINA

The vagina is a muscular, tube-shaped organ with an opening to the world (protected by the vulva) on one end and the cervix at the other. This is the pathway for babies and menstrual blood when they exit the uterus, and also the place where things are inserted, like a sex toy, finger, penis, tampon, or menstrual cup.

The walls of the vagina are sort of ruffled, covered with folds called rugae that allow it to expand and accommodate movement—like the folds that connect the two sections of an articulated bus. Vaginal tissue is layered and dynamic, moist with mucus on the surface but muscular and elastic directly beneath.

CERVIX

The cervix is the gatekeeper of the uterus! It's a short column of fibrous muscle with one side (the endocervix) open to the uterus and the other, nearly closed side (ectocervix), facing the vagina. The small opening on the vaginal side (called the os) is where sperm can enter and also the path out for menstrual blood and babies. With its capacity to both thin and stretch, the cervix can dilate a full ten centimeters. Cervical texture and tension morph throughout the menstrual cycle, and cervical fluids also vary in viscosity; this is how the cervix manages the traffic of bacteria and sperm into the uterus. These changes can be used in combination with other indicators to track where you are in your cycle, including when you're likely to be ovulating.

UTERUS

We know it as the place where babies and periods come from, but the uterus is also an important structural component in the pelvis. In its "resting" state, when it's not occupied, this organ is only about the size of a plum and weighs around two ounces. Anchored in place by ribbons of ligament running through the pelvis, the uterus helps keep the bladder and bowels in position. At its base is the cervix, and it connects to a fallopian tube on each side of its top.

The uterine wall, much like that of the vagina, is constantly changing. We'll talk more about that when we review the menstrual cycle.

FALLOPIAN TUBES

The fallopian tubes look like a pair of scrawny arms that come off the shoulders of the uterus. They arc out and down, as if draped around the neck of a buddy, with their open hands dangling right above the ovaries. The finger-like ends of each tube make a sweeping motion over the ovaries to catch matured eggs as they are released—think sea anemone. This movement ideally propels the egg through one of these four-inch tubes into the uterus.

OVARIES

Positioned on either side of the uterus, ovaries are held in place by ligaments, anchored to the pelvic wall above and to the uterus below. Each ovary comes into the world with about one million immature eggs, each encapsulated in a follicle. These eggs and follicles are minuscule, as the ovary itself is only about the size of a shelled almond. Ovaries are not only the star organs of the menopause show, but because they produce and release hormones, they are also considered one of the major glands in the endocrine system. Only one other organ in the body, the pancreas, shares this double-agent (organ and gland) distinction.

PELVIC BOWL

Our reproductive system is nestled between our hips, inside a bony structure called the pelvic bowl. It's woven like a basket with

WHAT IS MENOPAUSE?

ligaments and muscles. Reproductive organs are cradled by the group of muscles that make up the pelvic floor, at the base of the pelvic bowl. These muscles also support the bladder and rectum.

WHAT ARE HORMONES AND HOW DO THEY WORK?

We are going to talk a lot about hormones throughout this book because they are integral to the menopause transition and are one of your body's primary tools for communication between its systems and parts. Hormones are like the text messages of the body, and they are managed by your endocrine system, the network of glands that make and dispense hormones. If you've ever wondered how your body does just about anything it does without you thinking about it—grow, digest, heat up, stress out—the answer probably involves hormones. The glands in your endocrine system produce and release hormones into the bloodstream based on sensory information they get from hormone levels—yes, hormones sometimes control other hormones—and electronic pulses from your nervous system.

Because your blood travels through your entire body, it's impossible for your endocrine glands to send specific hormones directly to a specific cell or cells. Luckily, the cells in your body have receptors that allow substances to bind to them; each receptor is like a lock that only fits with certain kinds of keys (hormones are the keys). Once attached, the hormones can deliver instructions to start, stop, speed up, or slow down some kind of action in the receptor cell. So, endocrine glands can let hormones loose in your bloodstream because there are specific receptor cells, like little docking stations, waiting to receive them.

There are approximately fifty hormones in the human body, and they affect everything from growth and metabolism to immune response and fertility. Cortisol, insulin, and serotonin are all hormones you might be familiar with. Respectively, they regulate the stress response, metabolism, and mood. Sex hormones are the group of hormones that influence all activities in your reproductive system from development through retirement, but they also deliver instructions to many other systems throughout the body.

In addition to delivering information by connecting with receptor cells, hormones also influence activity in the body through mechanisms called *feedback loops,* which are regulatory processes amplifying or inhibiting activities with a goal of creating equilibrium in the body. Your body's internal systems are designed to function best when they are as close as possible to equilibrium or within a set acceptable range. The shared goal of all systems in the human body is *homeostasis,* which is the body's capacity to maintain stability within its internal systems. Our bodies never rest in a state of equilibrium because we are dynamic creatures, exerting ourselves through physical movement, eating and drinking, and being constantly stimulated by our environment (temperature, stress, lighting). Systems throughout the body are always making adjustments to keep things like internal temperature and blood sugar relatively stable as we go about our daily lives. Our bodies are responding to our surroundings and activities in every moment, even while we're sleeping. As you move through your day, even if you spend most of your day at a desk, your environment, actions, and reactions are forcing your body to work to maintain stability within your internal systems.

There are two main communication systems in your body that direct all cellular activity: nervous and endocrine. As we just learned, each of these systems has tools for sending out commands and instructions without talking; the nervous system uses electronic pulses and hormones, and the endocrine system uses hormones. Both of these tools are involved in feedback loops. There are two kinds of feedback loops: positive and negative. Positive feedback loops amplify change, negative feedback loops reduce change.

One of the easiest feedback loops to explain is the one your body uses to regulate temperature. We know that the ideal resting temperature for the body is around 98 degrees Fahrenheit. If your body temperature rises, the temperature of your blood does too, and your nervous system responds by shutting off heat-promoting activity and prompting skin blood vessels to dilate so that more blood will flow through them and release heat via the surface of your skin. Sweat glands are also activated to perspire, and those beads of sweat are vaporized by your body heat, which also cools your body. As your temperature comes down, your blood cools and your nervous system turns off your heat-loss center. This is a negative feedback loop because the product of the reaction—in this case, cooling—leads to a decrease in that reaction: your body stops sweating and dilating your blood vessels when you cool off.

Activities in your reproductive system are managed through a collection of feedback loops between your hypothalamus (part of your nervous system), your pituitary gland (part of your endocrine system), and your ovaries (part of your reproductive and endocrine systems). Here is an example of a negative feedback loop in your reproductive system: When the level of estrogen in your bloodstream drops, the hypothalamus sends a message (aka hormone) to the pituitary gland instructing it to release follicle stimulating hormone (FSH) into the bloodstream. FSH levels go up in your blood and connect with receptor cells in your ovaries. The increase in FSH prompts the ovaries to release estrogen into the bloodstream. Some of that estrogen stimulates activities in the ovary, such as maturing a follicle, but it also flows through the rest of the body, elevating the estrogen level in your blood. As this blood flows through the body, eventually reaching the hypothalamus, the hypothalamus senses elevated estrogen levels and stops sending messages to the pituitary to send FSH. As estrogen levels decline, the hypothalamus will start the process all over again by stimulating the pituitary.

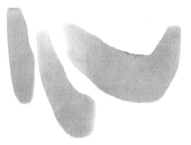

STAGES OF YOUR REPRODUCTIVE LIFE CYCLE

Physiological education in the classroom and doctor's office tends to focus on puberty and pregnancy. While this is understandable (because: babies), skimming over the rest of the cycle sends a message that it's somehow less interesting or important. In addition, most other information about the body is delivered on a "need to know" basis: unless you're having a problem or something changes significantly, you probably won't ever learn anything about it. But developmental changes in your body are a big deal, and knowledge is power.

Although understanding the physiology of your reproductive system does not change what's coming or what's already underway, it can offer a window onto the bigger picture that there will always be fluctuations in your body—a reminder that, for better or worse, things will always change.

PRE-MENSTRUATION

Let's begin at the beginning. If you are a cisgender woman or otherwise were assigned female at birth, you will likely have some combination of the following: two ovaries, two fallopian tubes, one uterus, one cervix, one vagina, and one vulva

At birth, each ovary holds one to two million microscopic immature egg cells. Each egg has the potential to achieve maturity, meet a sperm, and become an embryo. From birth on, the ovaries undergo a constant process of egg depletion. Between birth and the beginning of your transition through puberty, the number of eggs is reduced to just under half a million. The eggs nestled in those follicles cannot fully mature without the prodding of sex hormones, which your body doesn't produce until you enter puberty.

PUBERTY

Puberty is a hormonal transition that your body goes through, typically starting between ages eight and thirteen. Your reproductive system is ramping up to fertility and, like perimenopause, the process can be a bit destabilizing because a lot of change is happening in your body all at once.

Puberty begins when the hypothalamus, the pituitary gland, and the ovaries begin to communicate with each other. This invisible "line" of communication, which is actually a series of hormonal feedback loops, is called the HPO axis, and it is the way your body manages ovulation and menstruation. Like any new working relationship, it takes time for the H (hypothalamus), P (pituitary), and O (ovaries) to find a groove where everyone understands each other.

During the getting-to-know-you phase, there are some erratic hormone levels and intense experiences throughout the body as tissue and systems respond to sex hormones that they've never seen before: estrogen, progesterone, and testosterone. Everyone has all three sex hormones, but bodies with more estrogen and progesterone are typically designated female, while those with more testosterone are designated male. There are also intersex individuals (an estimated 1 to 2 of every 100 people born in the U.S.), who are born with sex hormone levels, genitals, and/or internal sex organs such that they are not designated male or female.

Scientists have not declared a definitive reason or trigger for the onset of puberty. It's tempting to imagine the ovaries patiently waiting for those sex hormones to show up, but research on animals shows that the ovaries might play a role in suppressing the gonadotrophin-releasing hormone (GnRH) released by the brain that would initiate puberty.

There is a long list of physical symptoms associated with puberty: acne, mood swings, body odor, and general growth spurts all over the body. During puberty estrogen and progesterone trigger breast development, widening of the hips, growth of pubic hair, vaginal discharge, and the beginning of ovulation and menstruation—the first menstrual bleed is called menarche. Any one of these changes would be a big deal, and having them all clustered together has the potential to feel overwhelming. In her book *The Body Is Not an Apology: The Power of Radical Self-Love*, activist Sonya Renee Taylor recalls what it felt like to be judged by the ways her body was developing: "From that moment forward, puberty became synonymous with public humiliation. I learned that our bodies and their changes were areas of public domain—and things to broadcast, be teased about, be ashamed of." Because you live in a body, you have experienced the ways that your physical form is an integral part of how others perceive you, which is one of the reasons that changes in our bodies can be so challenging.

One key difference between puberty and menopause is that the end of puberty is not defined by the arrival of the first menstrual period; that often comes around the halfway point. Because puberty is the process of readying the reproductive system, it is considered complete when breasts and genitalia are fully developed, pubic hair has grown in, and you've reached your full height. The ultimate marker of the completion of puberty is regular ovulatory cycles. At that point, your body is physiologically capable of reproducing and theoretically has the capacity to focus its energy on developing another human.

MENSTRUATION AND FERTILITY

Menstruation is the cycle of activity that readies your body each month (or so) for conceiving a child. Though we think of menstruation as one cycle, it's actually two interconnected tracks of activity. Track one is all about the work of the ovaries, and track two is focused on events happening in the uterus. Your sex hormones direct the activities in both tracks of your menstrual cycle. Estrogen and progesterone are the most well-known "female" sex hormones, but cisgender women produce small amounts of testosterone as well, at least one-tenth the amount that cisgender men produce. Three other hormones—FSH, luteinizing hormone, and GnRH—also play critical roles in your menstrual cycles. This chart shows you where these hormones are made and where they have influence (receptors) in your body.

HORMONE	PRODUCED BY	RECEPTORS IN
Estrogen (3 varieties: estradiol, estriol, estrone)	Ovaries, adrenal glands, fat tissue	Breasts, uterus, vulva, vagina, urinary tract, brain, bones, liver, heart, blood vessels, hair, mucous membranes, pelvic muscles, skin, gastrointestinal tract, eyes, skeletal and smooth muscles
Progesterone	Ovaries, adrenal glands, placenta (during pregnancy)	Uterus, ovaries, breasts, brain, thyroid, heart, bones, pancreas, urinary tract
Follicle-stimulating hormone (FSH)	Pituitary gland	Ovaries, uterus
Luteinizing hormone (LH)	Pituitary gland	Ovaries
Gonadotrophin-releasing hormone (GnRH)	Hypothalamus	Pituitary gland, ovaries, breasts
Testosterone	Ovaries, adrenal glands	Bones, kidneys, liver, muscles, ovaries, uterus, vagina, brain, blood vessels, heart

It's easiest to understand how these tracks of activity are interconnected if we walk through one full cycle. The cycle described in the following chart tracks the timeline of the "average" twenty-eight-day cycle. The design of early hormonal birth control in packets containing twenty-eight pills normalized this "average" cycle length, but it's important to note that each body has a unique cycle rhythm and corresponding length. When you first begin menstruating, your cycles can be variable and much longer because your reproductive system is still getting into the swing of things; it's not consistent right out of the gate. Over time, assuming you have a baseline of steady overall health, your cycle settles into a routine. Don't fret if the schedule outlined in this chart does not reflect your experience exactly. That said, if your cycles are inconsistent, infrequent, absent, shorter than twenty-one days (from day 1 of a cycle to day 1 of the next cycle), or longer than thirty-five days, it's a good idea to check in with a medical professional about it.

Here is the play-by-play for an "average" cycle:

MENSTRUAL CYCLE

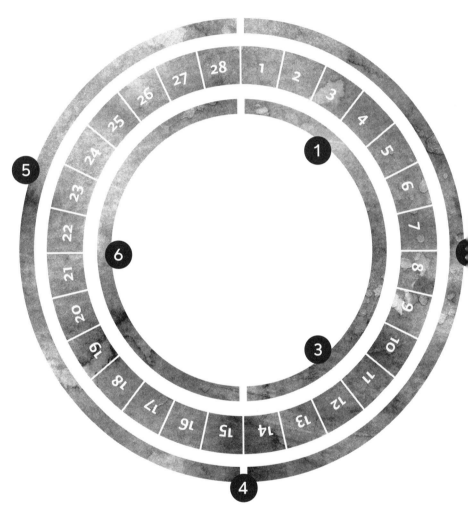

❶ MENSTRUAL FLOW (UTERINE TRACK)

Day 1 of your menstrual cycle is the first day you bleed. This phase, sometimes called menstrual flow, generally lasts three to five days, but can be as short as two and as long as seven days and still be considered normal.

❷ FOLLICULAR PHASE: DAYS 1–14 (OVARIAN TRACK)

Your ovaries notice an increase in FSH and begin maturing a handful of egg follicles. These first ten to fourteen days of the ovarian cycle are called the follicular phase because the main activity is the development of the sheath-like structure where eggs are matured, called a follicle. As follicles develop, they release estrogen—specifically estradiol. This phase can be as short as seven or as long as twenty-one days.

❸ BUILDING (UTERINE TRACK)

All the estrogen coming from the ovarian follicles cues the uterus to rebuild a thick, welcoming lining for potential visitors (aka fertilized eggs).

❹ OVULATION: DAY 14 (OVARIAN TRACK)

The midpoint of the ovarian cycle is ovulation—the release of a matured egg—which takes place immediately following the end of the follicular phase. The most mature follicle produces estrogen continually as it develops, and once the estrogen level is high enough, it triggers the hypothalamus to send out luteinizing hormone (LH). LH causes the mature follicle to rupture, allowing the egg to float out into the open arms of the fallopian tube. Short but sweet, it happens in a day.

❺ LUTEAL PHASE: DAYS 15–28 (OVARIAN TRACK)

The ruptured follicle that released a mature egg becomes a progesterone factory and distribution outlet called the corpus luteum. If the egg isn't fertilized, the corpus luteum eventually degenerates, halting the flow of progesterone and estrogen. This phase starts the day after ovulation and can be as short as ten or as long as sixteen days.

❻ DISMANTLING (UTERINE TRACK)

Around day 14, the hormones in your reproductive system shift, and the presence of progesterone (from the corpus luteum) tells uterine cells to stop thickening and begin secreting chemical messengers that get the lining ready for implantation. Unless a fertilized egg shows up, progesterone levels then decline drastically, cutting off the blood supply to the uterine wall, which eventually sheds as menstruation begins again.

It's a lot to take in, especially when most of us think of menstruation as a black box containing PMS, period blood, and the potential for pregnancy. In her book *Hormone Repair Manual: Every Woman's Guide to Healthy Hormones after 40*, naturopath Lara Briden writes, "You may have been given the impression that menstrual cycles are only for making babies and that, once you're done with all that, you can take or leave periods. In reality, menstrual cycles are not just for making babies; they're also for making hormones." As we explore the transition to menopause you will learn about all the influence estrogen and progesterone have in systems throughout your body. Understanding the value of these hormones might change how you look at your menstrual cycle, the role it plays in your overall health, and why your body feels it when these cycles become irregular and eventually stop at menopause.

Knowing what's happening in your body might also make it more interesting to track your cycle (fertility awareness isn't only for people focused on pregnancy!), something we will explore more in part three.

Is Your Menstrual Cycle a Vital Sign?

Menstruation is being destigmatized. We're not there yet, but people around the world are working hard to break down period taboos. The work of this movement is happening at the same time that the medical establishment is beginning to consider the menstrual cycle to be a fifth vital sign. Vital signs show us the state of our essential body functions, and they are the indicators doctors use to assess wellness. The four primary vital signs standard in most medical settings are body temperature, pulse rate, respiration rate, and blood pressure.

Viewing the menstrual cycle as a marker of health rather than a discrete aspect of a singular function of our bodies (reproduction) is a paradigm shift, a fundamental change in our understanding of the body. It takes time for a change like this to work its way through both our minds and the systems we've built around what we used to believe. Our healthcare system hasn't hesitated to suppress women's reproductive functions (often with hormonal contraception) at the first sign of symptoms perceived to be caused by the reproductive system like acne, heavy or absent periods, or ovarian cysts. Hormonal contraception is a powerful tool that can quite literally transform an individual's quality of life by addressing any of the issues I just mentioned and giving people agency of their reproductive lives. It's true that hormonal contraception is a powerful tool—I do not want to diminish that power—but I do want to consider what it costs us.

Nuance is the first thing to go in discussions about the uterus. Because of the positive and powerful aspects of hormonal contraception, criticism of it is often seen as unfriendly to the reproductive equity movement. And yet, as Lisa Hendrickson-Jack notes in her book *The Fifth Vital Sign: Master Your Cycles and Optimize Your Fertility*, "Enovid [the first hormonal birth control pill] was the first drug ever developed to shut down a perfectly normal bodily function in healthy individuals." The fear of losing any contraceptive ground can keep us from demanding knowledge, treatment modalities, and even pharmaceuticals that offer us agency without sacrificing a normal bodily function.

So many who menstruate learn only to fear pregnancy and dread periods because we don't learn enough to understand all that happens through our cycles. I had never thought my period could tell me much of anything beyond whether or not I was pregnant. However, the menstrual cycle is an additional vital sign for those with ovaries and a uterus—a line of communication with our bodies that is there waiting to share information with us. If you're interested in deciphering the signals your body is sending through your cycle, there are a few great books and many dedicated practitioners (see the Resources section) that can help you.

PERIMENOPAUSE

The path to retirement looks different for every ovary, just like it does for people. For most, though, it is not a decline with a steady or predictable pitch; it's more likely to be filled with ups and downs.

Perimenopause is the time your body spends transitioning from menstruation and fertility to menopause—the beginning of your post-reproductive years, when you no longer have periods and can no longer conceive or carry a baby. The specific forces that initiate perimenopause are murky, but we do know that during this phase of your reproductive life span your ovaries are slowly retiring from their primary functions: maturing and releasing eggs. However, if your ovaries are surgically removed or impacted by a chemical treatment like chemotherapy that stops them from maturing and releasing eggs, you immediately enter menopause. If you weren't in perimenopause at the time of your procedure, this kind of abrupt transition will require your body to make an equally abrupt adjustment to the lower levels of sex hormones. Otherwise, the perimenopause transition unfolds over time, anywhere from two to ten years.

As we learned earlier, menstrual cycles are managed through feedback loops along the HPO axis. During perimenopause, every part of the axis becomes less sensitive and, as a result, less responsive—like when one finicky bulb makes an entire strand of holiday lights flicker. When messaging frequency and intensity fluctuate, all the cells in the body with receptors for estrogen or progesterone are impacted. At a pace determined by a multitude of factors—genetics, environmental influences, lived experiences—the ovaries become progressively less responsive to the hormonal messages that used to launch them into action. Your ovaries slow down in part because your follicles (the sheaths that house developing eggs) decline in quality and number as you age and also because they become less sensitive to the arrival of FSH from the pituitary. As a result, they don't release as much estrogen. Without the boost of estrogen, eggs don't fully mature, and follicles don't rupture. If follicles don't rupture to release an egg, there is no release of progesterone. Declining progesterone is associated with some of the symptoms of perimenopause, such as heavier periods, shorter cycles, disrupted sleep, and breast tenderness.

In addition, estrogen can spike at times when the ovaries respond to the FSH that the pituitary continues to send in absence of a message from the ovaries telling it to stop. During perimenopause, there are times when estrogen levels can be up to three times higher than before. High estrogen levels do not guarantee ovulation during perimenopause—because the follicles are older and their quality is lower—and this means that there might not be any progesterone released to help offset or mitigate the effects of high estrogen.

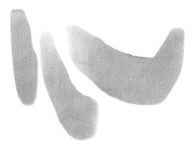

WHAT IS MENOPAUSE?

The Language of Menopause

The language used by doctors—ovarian failure, follicular exhaustion, vaginal atrophy—to describe what the body does and doesn't do during perimenopause and at menopause is harsh and, at times, verges on ridiculous. One woman I interviewed shared that when she asked her doctor if she was menopausal, now that she had gone eleven months without a period, her doctor replied, "No, you haven't achieved successful ovarian failure yet." The absurdity of that statement makes me laugh every time I think of it, but the negative connotations of words like *failure, exhaustion,* and *atrophy* can have harmful effects on us.

As much as we may consider medical terminology to be objective because it is within the realm of science, language is rarely neutral, especially when it is exchanged between people in a specific context, like you and your practitioner discussing your health. Medical professionals may think that referring to menopause as an estrogen deficiency is simply stating the reality of a person's endocrinology, but the word *deficiency* implies a lacking or shortage of something, which categorizes what's happening in your body as a problem. An evolutionary biologist may take issue with this suggestion of menopause as a deficient state because it implies a malfunction instead of a change that is evidence of an adaptation or a shift in reproductive strategy. An individual going through the menopause transition might be confused by the word *deficiency* because the doctor keeps telling them that this transition is *natural*.

Perimenopause is accurately described as *natural* and *normal* by medical professionals and older women alike, and while true, our positive associations with these words can also conflict with the

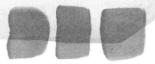

reality of our experience. *Natural* and *normal* don't mean that something will be easy, better, or gentle, but these words can make people feel like they shouldn't be struggling in this transition or that, if they are, then something is wrong with them.

Doctors and researchers are not the only ones constructing our understanding of menopause. The media (including me), companies, and academics contribute to meaning-making too. In her 1995 essay "More Than the Change: Diversity and Flexibility in Menopausal Experience" published in *Hot Flashes: Women Writers on the Change of Life*, anthropological researcher Denise Spitzer outlines four explanatory models of menopause: medical, sociocultural, vulnerability, self-help. Each model uses specific language to create a unique description and constellation of meaning around menopause. Spitzer summarizes the various models this way: "menopause is a disease, a cultural phenomenon without reference to biology, an indicator of stress, or a time for self and celebration." All these models have persisted, which is one of the reasons why we hear conflicting descriptions and vocabularies of menopause.

"I really didn't know what to expect. I think that people talk about women getting really irritable in menopause or cycles stopping, you can no longer conceive. I watched older women in my life and would be like, *Why are they wearing comfortable shoes, and why are they cutting their hair short, and why are they gaining weight around the middle?* It all [felt] kind of far away then. It's a hell of a lot closer now." —AIMEE

Simply put, during perimenopause the same hormones that flooded your system in puberty are fluctuating before they ultimately taper off. The changes or symptoms you experience are evidence of your body's attempting to adjust to these new levels. If you drink one cup of regular coffee every day, your body gets used to that daily dose of caffeine. Imagine that you decide to switch to herbal tea cold turkey; your body will probably have a response to the lack of caffeine, such as a headache or a dip in your energy level. Now let's imagine that your coffee habits go through a less predictable transition, as perimenopause does. One morning you drink four cups, the next day eight, followed by none on the third day. Like the effects of shifting hormone levels in perimenopause, this caffeine chaos would play out differently in individual bodies; it might send some people running for the toilet or grabbing for a bottle of headache reliever, while others might feel a little jittery but otherwise be okay.

"Common"
Perimenopause Symptoms

There is debate about how this list of symptoms has been developed and the ways in which it has been reinforced by medical and media professionals. Anthropologists, sociologists, historians, and feminists have all documented the inconsistency of symptoms reporting and data collection around the world. The symptoms and experiences listed below are the ones that Western culture generally accepts as "common" during perimenopause. To be clear, commonality does not mean universality; you may experience one, some, or none of them in your transition. We will review these symptoms and more in chapter 3.

Hot flashes and night sweats

Disrupted sleep

Changes to menstrual cycle

Brain fog, cognitive changes, memory loss

Vaginal discomfort—itching, burning, pain with penetration

Change in interest in sex and sexual function

Urinary incontinence, increased frequency or urgency

Body composition changes

Thinning hair

Dry skin

Anxiety

Depression

Joint pain

Perimenopause is a time when many people feel like their body is gaslighting them. The HPO axis seems to have developed a mind of its own; some weeks it sticks to the familiar routine and others it drops the ball entirely. Menstrual cycles—and all the accompanying activities you associate with your cycle—can vacillate wildly or modestly between over- and underfunctioning. This can look like changes in your cycle length (longer or shorter), the volume and duration of bleeding each cycle, and new experiences like vaginal dryness. The timing of perimenopause for many women (midlife) only adds to the body's homeostasis workload because it coincides with the early stages of aging and other demands of adult life like career and family.

Note that there is research showing that, when experienced in midlife, the transition to menopause does not consistently take center stage in women's lives because of all the other competing demands of this time. A qualitative research study conducted in the mid-aughts by Dr. Heather Dillaway, a sociologist focusing on women's experiences of menopause and midlife, set out to understand the variety of ways that menopause is experienced by a diverse group of women. In "Talking 'Among Us': How Women from Different Racial-Ethnic Groups Define and Discuss Menopause," Dillaway and her coauthors Mary Byrnes, Sara Miller, and Sonica Rehan report that Black participants "often implied that more important problems, for instance, other health or aging conditions or family problems, needed their time, energy and resources; thus menopause (and their feelings about its potentially never-ending nature) had to fall to the wayside." Dillaway noted that the less intense focus on menopause reported by Black women in her study was not the result of less awareness of the bodily transition they were going through, nor an indication of the quantity or severity of their symptoms; rather, it was a difference influenced by cultural forces and potentially class differences as well.

More recent research that draws on data from the U.S. Study of Women's Health Across the Nation (SWAN), a decades-long research study of the health of midlife women across ethnicities, also points to socioeconomic differences as significant factors in an individual's experience of the menopause transition, both in terms of physiology and quality-of-life ratings.

MENOPAUSE

Technically, menopause is a moment: it is the one-year anniversary of your final menstrual period, the marker of the end of your fertility. Arrival at menopause does not mean anything more than that your ovaries have fully retired from ovulation. Any symptoms you have been experiencing during perimenopause won't automatically stop along with your periods, though it does appear that many of them do decline and often disappear within the first year or two after menopause.

POSTMENOPAUSE

There isn't nearly as much enthusiasm in the media for discussing this phase of menopause, because it touches the territory of aging. Physiologically speaking, sex hormone levels are relatively stable in postmenopause because ovulation hasn't happened in at least a year and the HPO axis has found a new, steadier groove. That said, cells throughout the body that received instructions from estrogen (or progesterone or testosterone) will function differently when they don't have access to as much of it or, in some cases, to the same type of hormone.

While you were fertile and ovulating, your ovaries mainly produced estradiol, the strongest form of estrogen with the longest staying power at receptor cells. After menopause, your body will rely more on another form of estrogen, called estrone, which is produced by your ovaries, adrenal glands, and adipose fat tissue. When estrogen production in your ovaries plummets, the impact is twofold: lower levels of estrogen overall in the body and a shift in the dominant form of estrogen from a strong one (estradiol) to a weaker one (estrone). Lower estrogen levels of a less potent form are but one contributing factor to the increased risk of decline in bone density and cardiovascular health. The way your body ages will also be influenced by numerous other factors beyond the retirement of your ovaries, such as stress, genetics, lifestyle, and environment.

Symptoms of perimenopause, like hot flashes and headaches, decline for most people in the first couple of years postmenopause, but it is possible that they will persist longer. Even if symptoms persist, it is possible to continue to enjoy life in all the ways you do today, albeit possibly with some modifications to relationships, physical exercise, sex, and intellectual pursuits. If you're experiencing menopause in midlife, the other major influences during the postmenopausal years are the physical changes associated with normal aging and the implications of living within a culture in which negative ideas about aging and older people are entrenched. Experiencing these biases, in addition to others you may face in response to other components of your identity, can have very a real impact on your mental and physical health over time.

WHY DO WE GO THROUGH MENOPAUSE?

Not many species live beyond their reproductive years, especially not mammals. Author Darcey Steinke captivated readers when she explored her feeling of kinship with killer whales, one of the few other mammals we know of that go through menopause, in her book *Flash Count Diary: Menopause and the Vindication of Natural Life*. Many of the people going through menopause I spoke with in my research guessed that menopause is a relatively new human experience, because our life expectancy has gone up and we are living longer after our reproductive years. Although there may be a hint of truth in this idea (we do live more post-reproductive years than our ancestors), it misses an important question: is menopause an adaptive trait that was part of our evolution? The answer to this question has implications for the way we see menopause, both medically and culturally. Presuming that menopause is just a byproduct of our longer life spans implies at best that menopause holds little to no evolutionary benefit and at worst that menopause is a problematic breakdown of the body.

While it seems counter to evolutionary logic that female humans would live beyond their reproductive years, researchers in the 1960s developed a theory about why menopause makes evolutionary sense. Rather than continuing to make more offspring, post-reproductive females become providers of resources—food, care, expertise—for their offspring's children. Ultimately, if their children have more children that survive, their genes not only persist but persist in larger numbers. The crux of the Grandmother Hypothesis, as this leading theory is known, is the idea that, with the additional support of post-reproductive females, women can start having children earlier and more frequently, and that those children will have better survival odds.

Most evolutionary biology theories acknowledge menopause as adaptive rather than accidental. In her book *The Slow Moon Climbs: The Science, History, and Meaning of Menopause*, historian Susan P. Mattern considers multiple theories that illuminate the value of a lengthening post-reproductive life span. She outlines how menopause fits as an adaptive reproductive strategy in the most prominent theories of evolutionary biology, and how it continues to serve us in the modern world because it keeps the ratio of people who are reproducing and people who are not reproducing (and ideally providing help) in some degree of balance.

There is a long history of scientists attempting to explain the inner workings of female reproductive physiology, often from the apparent perspective that its processes, organs, and parts need to be managed or controlled. Although it's difficult to quantify how much, it is hard to deny that scientific theories and medical research have the power to influence the ways we experience changes in our bodies. Would your experience of menopause be different if you believed, for example, that each person designated female at birth was born with a certain allotment of menstrual blood and that menopause simply marked the end of their supply? The value of this kind of question is not in the answer but in the way it reminds us that, like all other physiological processes (birth, death, etc.), menopause is—and has always been—both a physiological experience and a cultural construct.

THE MENOPAUSAL MILIEU

Just like a plant is impacted greatly by the place where its planted, the environment you live in influences you physically and emotionally. The place where you live is but one of the facets that compose your environment. Physical elements (air, water, landscape, and built environments like houses or offices), cultural and societal components (belief systems, civic structures, food traditions, and relationships), and your economic situation (which often has implications for the physical and cultural and societal aspects of your environment) all directly influence the person you become in body and spirit. Your ability to control your environment fluctuates over the course of your lifetime, according to structural and systemic biases in your culture, your socioeconomic status within a fluctuating economy, and in accordance with specific choices that you make or that are made for you.

YOUR PHYSICAL ENVIRONMENT

What does where you live have to do with your reproductive and overall health? A lot. A high-profile example of this is the mismanaged lead toxicity in the public water supply that negatively impacted the health of an entire generation of children in Flint, Michigan. You may remember a lot of loud concerns in the late aughts about additives in plastics with names like bisphenols (BPA) and phthalates that had potentially harmful effects on tissues throughout the human body. Researchers were, and still are, exploring exactly how these chemical compounds interact with cells in various parts of our bodies. In both instances—lead in the water supply and chemicals in plastics—not everyone who is exposed to these substances is impacted in the same way. Part of that is about the level of exposure to toxins, but genetics probably plays a role too, along with the overall health of each individual prior to their exposure. Various environmental toxins have been (and continue to be) studied in relation to women's health issues including reproductive cancers, endometriosis, and infertility.

What's an Endocrine Disruptor?

When you are out in the world, various cells make their way into your body through things you eat, drink, breathe, or absorb through your skin. Some of these cells from outside of your body fit perfectly in receptor cells inside your body, and if they latch on, they can either deliver information (just like hormones produced within your body would) or block your hormones from attaching to their receptor cells. Either way, they disrupt functions of the endocrine system, which is why they're called endocrine disruptors.

Most of the information we hear about endocrine disruptors in the news or from doctors is focused the endocrine-disrupting chemicals and compounds found in things like plastics that we use to package food as well as in household products, pesticides, insecticides, and herbicides. Some of these manufactured endocrine disruptors have been banned because of documented negative health effects. Endocrine disruptor research identifies ways that these cells negatively affect reproduction, metabolism, and neurological function and cause cancers. Messages in the media about detoxifying your home often include advice about limiting your exposure to endocrine disruptors found in fabrics, household cleaners, food containers, home improvement products, and pesticides and herbicides.

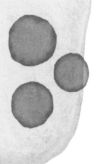

WHAT IS MENOPAUSE?

Exposure to any toxin, regardless of whether it is by choice—as in smoking or drug use—or at the hand of another—via pollution or household products—does not guarantee negative health outcomes, but it does increase your risk of a list of potential problems and diseases. The way doctors encourage us to think about it is that each time we are exposed to some thing or environment known to be challenging for our body, like a loud concert or a polluted lake, we increase our risk of negative outcomes in our health. Situated in midlife for many, the menopause transition is influenced considerably by the cumulative effects of exposure to harmful environmental factors over the course of one's lifetime.

THE CULTURE YOU LIVE IN

Culture can influence health outcomes in myriad ways. The effects of diet and specific culinary traditions on health have been well documented for decades—who hasn't heard about the virtues of the Mediterranean diet? There is also evidence that specific foods that are ingrained in a culture's culinary traditions have health implications, such as the studies showing that high consumption of phytoestrogen-rich tofu in the Japanese diet may reduce certain symptoms during the menopausal transition.

Beliefs and norms can also influence behaviors that ultimately affect health. In the U.S. we have only just begun to collectively examine and reckon with the white supremacist roots of our culture. There are numerous studies capturing the harm of systemic racism to the mental and physical health of Black and Brown Americans. The Center for Disease Control data on the Black maternal mortality rate (2.5 times the rate of non-Hispanic white women, and 3.5 times the rate of Hispanic women) and the disproportionate number of COVID-19 deaths in communities of color are a couple of recent examples of racial disparities in health outcomes. Larger reviews, called meta-analyses, examining hundreds of research studies over previous decades have confirmed evidence that the effects of structural racism have a direct and negative effect on health outcomes for non-white Americans.

Relationships in your personal and professional life have the potential to directly influence your behaviors. If you hang out with a crew that's into CrossFit, you're likely to work out more often. If you're around a lot of people who like to stay out late, you will probably get less sleep. Any type of relationship—familial, friend, romantic, professional—has some effect on your emotions, maybe even elevating or lowering your stress level. Caregiving is a common role among people in the midst of perimenopause, whether it is for their children, parents, or other community members. Although caregiving can be rewarding and fulfilling, it is an investment of time and energy that adds emotional and logistical stress to your life.

In addition to the effects of the culture at large on your life are those from the micro-culture of your family, both genetically and environmentally. Research has demonstrated the impacts of trauma on the physical health of not only individuals who experience it but also their children. This phenomenon is called *intergenerational trauma*, and those at the highest risk are in families with a member who has experienced a significant form of abuse, neglect, and oppression, such as a survivor of genocide, war, displacement, and slavery.

YOUR SOCIOECONOMIC SITUATION

Lack of economic security and outright poverty are also associated with higher stress levels and negative mental and physical health outcomes. Research shows a clear relationship between poverty and an increased risk for chronic conditions, disease, and premature death. The impacts of economic inequity, and the accompanying lack of parity in access to resources, are also evident throughout menopause research, which cites low socioeconomic standing and low educational attainment as risk factors for symptoms like depression, metabolic disorders, and vasomotor symptoms (hot flashes and night sweats).

Stress and Your Cycle

"Stress" is the term we commonly use to describe a short- or long-term situation that makes us feel overwhelmed, tired, scared, or anxious. These feelings can be caused by environmental changes (moving, starting or losing a job, travel), physical changes (a brush with danger, illness, intense exercise), or emotional pressures (final exams, a breakup, the death of a loved one). Big changes, even the ones we make intentionally and feel great about, tend to be stressful.

In addition to our emotional experience, we also experience a physiological reaction to stress. You've probably heard about the ways our stress response evolved to protect us from harm by focusing our body's energy and resources on the systems required for us to survive life-threatening situations. When you experience persistent or chronic stress, the survival mechanisms in the body that were designed to provide short-term emergency assistance instead generate negative health impacts over time. Menstruation, along with digestion, metabolism, sleep, and even your immune response, can all be dysregulated by chronic stress.

Hormones released during the stress response can alter reproductive hormone activity, disrupting regular ovulation and resulting in skipped or irregular periods. As researcher and neuroscientist Lisa Mosconi explains in her TED Talk "How Menopause Affects the Brain," stress can influence estrogen levels in your body: cortisol goes up, estrogen goes down. Your body relies on sex hormones to manage processes in your reproductive system, but also to perform functions in other critical organs and tissues. Changes in your menstrual cycle can serve as a barometer of your overall health or, at the very least, do the job of a canary in a coal mine. Remember that hormonal birth control obscures your body's natural cycles and makes it much harder to assess how they are impacted by stress.

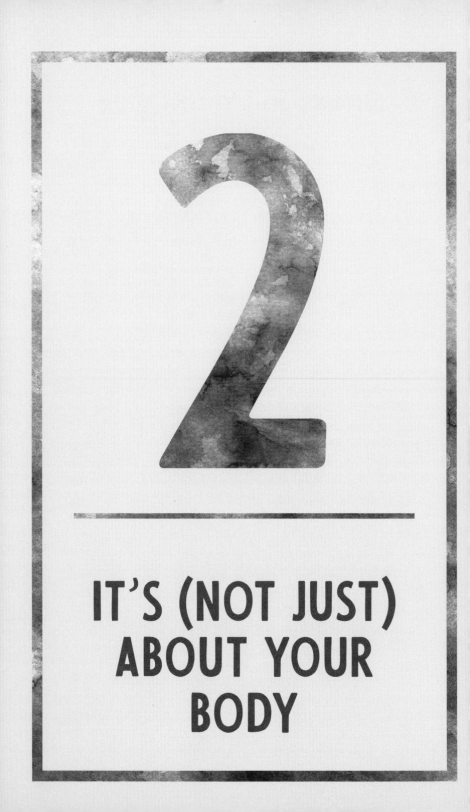

2

IT'S (NOT JUST) ABOUT YOUR BODY

Your understanding of and relationship to *your body* is fundamentally different from the scientific understanding of *the body*. *Your body* is where you live, how you do things, and a large part of your identity. *The body* is a group of interconnected systems hanging on a collection of bones and wrapped in a skin suit. *Your body* has the potential for achieving dreams and experiencing untold pleasures and pains. *The body* is a series of risk/benefit calculations. *Your body* encounters *the body* anytime you seek information, care, or expertise about your menopause experience.

Menopause is a bodily event, and it's also a shift in the ways you and your body experience and interact with the world. This makes it both an experience you live through, inside of *your body*—with real physical challenges such as insomnia, heavy bleeding, and memory loss—and an experience that is lived out in other contexts: medical, public, and intimate. In addition, the way that menopause is perceived and experienced is influenced by the pressures of modern capitalism and popular culture.

The interplay among these forces during the menopause transition is akin to the "three-body problem," an unsolvable mathematical quandary in which the trajectories of three celestial bodies cannot be accurately predicted because the movement of each body is governed by the influence of the others. In other words, the entanglement of multiple bodies makes it impossible to predict how each will move, let alone affect the others' movement. The three *bodies* at the center of the menopause conundrum are the personal, the cultural, and the political. "Political" here refers not to any specific government or official but more generally to structures of power in our society and the institutions that uphold them.

A change in any one of these bodies has a ripple effect through the others (including your own body). Each decision you make, explanation you get, and product or service you purchase, and the way you feel throughout the transition, is bound up in these interrelated forces. In addition to the variations in physiological symptoms it causes, this dynamic interplay can make menopause less like a clearly defined phenomenon and more like a shape-shifting wind that can gently breeze through one person's life but can touch down like a tornado in another's.

"I think one of the biggest things that needed to have happened is me being taught to love my body from the very beginning. That's the thing: being present in my body, being taught about the external pressures that are just on the daily from twelve years old on. You know, how I look, what I wear, my body, what I eat, what I say, how I have sex, who I have it with, how I do this thing, how I hate on myself, all that stuff. I don't think it's just necessarily talking about the event [menopause]; it's about having a life lived with genuine self-compassion. Self-compassion is love, it's having community, it's having connection, it's having an understanding of what's happening in our bodies from a very young age and learning how to negotiate our nervous systems and our fears and being open to our anxieties." —SARA

WHAT IS MENOPAUSE?

POLITICAL: YOUR BODY + THE BODY

There is no shortage of discussion about women's health in our society. Many of those conversations are centered around reproduction itself: pregnancy, the sex required to create said pregnancy, and birth. Viewing the body through the lens of reproduction influences everything from how women's health issues are prioritized to the questions researchers pose and study and which problems product developers attempt to address. In other words, the lens we look through determines not only what's in focus but also how we think about and interact with it.

A thorough examination of the female body throughout the history of medicine is well beyond the scope of this book. If you are interested in going deeper into the subject of sexism and racism in the field of medicine, you will find a list of incredible books authored by historians, researchers, and science journalists in the Resources section. Here we are going to focus on what it might be like for you—an individual in the midst of your menopause transition—as you interact with a couple of major structures of power in our society: the medical establishment and capitalism.

HOW DID WE GET HERE?

In her book *Everybody: A Book about Freedom*, Olivia Laing beautifully articulates the distance between the bodily perception of an individual and that of a medical professional. Laing is a trained herbalist who ran her own practice and years ago observed that her patients did not draw hard lines between their physical and emotional experiences. In their accounts, the upheavals of life events—moves, deaths, relationship shifts—were connected to the health issues they experienced. By comparison, some of the practitioners whom she had studied under perceived the body as definitively dissociated from personhood. To them events or changes in the body were mere functions or malfunctions of what amounted to machinery.

If you've ever had an examination with a practitioner in the Western medical system, the kind where, wearing a tragically thin cotton or paper smock slit up the front, you situate yourself atop a sheet of white paper at one end of a padded rectangular table, then you've probably experienced the sense of disconnect, or possibly the collision, between the two perspectives Laing is describing. Maybe it felt like you and your physician were speaking different languages as the details of your experience—achy joints, not feeling like myself, bleeding erratically—were translated into a different vocabulary—myalgia, mental health, amenorrhea—so they could be measured against metrics that were unfamiliar to you. Modern medical environments can feel like another planet populated by people speaking another language.

Science—the practice of and our belief in—cannot be disentangled from culture, because at its core science is a means of explaining our world using the tools we have at a given moment in time. Scientific knowledge, particularly the kind that explains how things like our bodies work, is power. Throughout most of history that particular power—medicine—was primarily the purview of cisgender, heterosexual white men who served at the pleasure of other, more powerful men. Unfortunately, these men generally perceived women's bodies as deviant or faulty versions of their own bodies. And because women were not permitted to speak for themselves, their bodies and experiences were filtered through the perceptions of men.

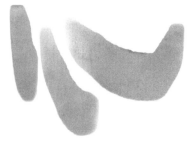

"So many of women's issues are [treated] like, *Oh yeah, that's happening. Okay. Next!* There's really not more said, and it's sort of a joke. Like, *They're having cramps,* or *They're having menopause,* or whatever it is—*you're hormonal*—and I think that gets wrapped up with age. There's a lot of, *Are you doing your Kegels?* and that feels like a simplification, maybe." —**KRISTIN**

Medical experts from ancient to modern times have always been entangled with societal power structures. Though community medicine has persisted throughout history in the form of midwives, witches, folk healers, homeopaths, and other alternative practitioners, ruling institutions—whether familial, religious, financial, or political—have influenced and governed medical beliefs and practices from the very beginning. Even after the institutions of medicine (universities, research facilities, doctor's offices, and hospitals) allowed women to participate, the institutions governing medicine (medical boards, politicians, and philanthropists) were still led and ruled by men. Mostly white men.

Although menstruation and fertility were always subjects of great interest to these men (both are thoroughly described in the earliest historical medical documents from ancient Greece and China), they did not inspire anything like reverence in Western doctrines. On the contrary, they were perceived as a considerable bother, because the female body and mind were already positioned as inferior to their male counterparts. Femaleness itself was a receptacle for blame. Whether it was due to a "wandering womb" or the lack of sufficient sexual interaction with a male phallus, the ancient Egyptians, Greeks,

and Romans all agreed that whatever problem was happening in a woman's body was the result of its inferior design. These ideas persisted through the Middle Ages and the Renaissance: women are perceived less as patients to be cured than as the causes of their own physical ailments.

It's not until the sixteenth century that the attention of practitioners and philosophers shifted from the uterus to the mind and nerves. "Hysteria" became a diagnostic umbrella for any unacceptable behaviors or health conditions of women that were difficult to explain. The notion of women having delicate minds and nerves provided sturdy scaffolding for the ideas about female weakness and fragility that kept women and girls out of education and the workforce. Miraculously, throughout the centuries, the treatments recommended for most women's ailments remained the same: marriage, sex, and childbearing.

For centuries, medical experts asserted that *all* diseases or discomforts experienced by women who had stopped menstruating were caused by a buildup of excess menstrual blood.

The regular release of menses was understood to be important to maintaining balance among the body's fluids and also to releasing the toxins believed to exist within menstrual blood. These beliefs about the purpose and composition of menstrual blood brought about the perception that the end of menstruation was the beginning of the end for a woman's health. Physicians were writing papers and books diagnosing and treating symptoms and illnesses associated with the end of menstruation (some accurately, others not) as early as the sixteenth century. The term *menopause* was not created until 1812, in a dissertation by French physician Dr. Charles Pierre Louis Gardanne. Naming menopause made it more visible within the medical profession and among the public, offering a framework to discuss the physiological changes in women's bodies clustered around the end of fertility and menstruation. Medical professionals did not agree about the meaning of menopause: negative associations about its impact on women's physical health and status were in the mix from the very beginning, but so were voices declaring that it was a natural course of change in the body.

The discovery of hormones in 1900 marked the beginning of the field of endocrinology, which led to our understanding of sex-specific hormones, including estrogen, progesterone, and testosterone. The underlying conceit that the very nature of women's bodies was a problem remained, but now the medical establishment came to believe the problem was caused by hormonal deficiency. Practitioners began prescribing hormones for relief of menopause symptoms in the early twentieth century, and by the 1950s hormones and sedatives were frequently prescribed to and requested by women with access to medical care. Note that throughout this time period, women with greater access to doctors and medicine were predominantly white and middle- or upper-class. Medicine's understanding of women's reproductive system evolved out of the "toxic menses" phase and into the hormonal phase. It's an interesting combination of ideas, right? On the one hand, there is this long history documenting that this is what women's bodies naturally do over time, and on the other, there is a persistent pressure on women to control their unruly bodies.

In her book *The Slow Moon Climbs: The Science, History, and Meaning of Menopause*, historian Susan P. Mattern unpacks how the inherent bias that women are inferior to men was perpetuated through cultural and medical responses to menopause throughout the twentieth century. If women did something that was considered unacceptable like "not doing housework, fighting with husbands, engaging in enthusiastic or promiscuous sex," hormones were deemed the culprit. These ideas about how women should look and act fueled the market for prescription hormones to bring the unruly body back in line. Prescription hormone therapy did offer many women relief from burdensome symptoms, but the problematic gender bias that was deeply embedded in the medical establishment's assessment and diagnosis of women's natural cycles did not.

The medical history of menopause cannot be separated from cultural shifts in perceptions about the role of women in society. Judith A. Houck documents just how entangled these histories are in her book *Hot and Bothered: Women, Medicine, and Menopause in Modern America*. Houck captures the way that the forces of medicine and culture constantly overlap and fold in on one another: "The history of menopause demonstrates that medicalization is not an endpoint but a process that responds over time to cultural pressures and technological developments. As the medical tools, players, and theories shift against a changing cultural backdrop, the content and reach of medicine similarly changes."

As the way women engage in public life changes, the expectations of women and practitioners shift, and this in turn leads to new and different perceptions of menopause for women and practitioners. This interwoven narrative of menopause is ever-evolving, which is probably why the sense of mystery remains. Our collective understanding, experience, and management of menopause will continue to evolve in this way for the duration of human existence. Although the physiology of menopause is unchanged from those first documented medical observations, the lived experience of menopause is different because we (as a collective and individuals) are all different.

WHY IS THERE STILL SO MUCH WE DON'T KNOW?

Medical practitioners and researchers within the medical field are not immune to the biases, -isms, or phobias of the day, because they swim in the same cultural and capitalistic tides as the patients they treat and the subjects they study. Throughout history, explanations of menopause have been extensions of the reigning—often bonkers!—theories of female physiology, which have unsurprisingly clustered consistently around themes of inferiority, frailty, and instability.

Practitioners and researchers actively did not listen to women for centuries. Though there have been shifts in the cultural and medical tides with respect to women and menopause, we're still in murky waters. Caroline Criado Perez, author of *Invisible Women: Data Bias in a World Designed for Men*, discovered that a survey of medical school textbooks that was conducted less than twenty years ago revealed that medical students still learn about "physiology" and "anatomy" followed by female physiology and female anatomy. Learning about the female body as a variation on the "standard" male body creates a sense of hierarchy where there isn't one. That hierarchy informs what garners attention, and dollars, in clinical practice and research.

Criado Perez notes women are excluded from medical research as a result of perceptions that their bodies and lives are overly complicated—by menstrual cycles, pregnancy, or seemingly inflexible schedules due to caregiving responsibilities. Leaving women out of research isn't only unfair, it's also dangerous, because our bodies are different from men's in ways that impact health outcomes beyond our reproductive systems, like the way female bodies often metabolize drugs differently than male bodies. When women are not included in research or studied independently, it perpetuates the current reality where there is no cache of historical data for comparison and thus no means of furthering our understanding of health challenges or outcomes in female bodies over time. Data is a major tool for drug (and other) companies to assess the market for new products; if they cannot see the challenges women face, like those resulting from endometriosis, autoimmune diseases, or menopause, they are less likely to develop products that offer relief from them. Clinical tools used by nurses and doctors to assess and diagnose patients are also built on data collected by researchers who have hardly ever considered all bodies—different sexes, shapes, sizes, races—in their studies.

Perceptions of specific medical conditions or health outcomes also impact the way research studies are structured and conducted and ultimately affect the quality of care given. It's easier to gather and assess quantitative data based on questions like "Which menopause symptoms are you experiencing? Check all that apply," followed by a laundry list of known symptoms than data from questions like "What has menopause been like for you?" The open-ended question might not yield comparable data, but it offers a range of responses that might include complaints about as yet undocumented symptoms and information about the variety of ways the menopause transition impacts someone's lifestyle, work, and relationships. It's the difference between someone checking the yes box next to "hot flashes" and telling you, as a woman I interviewed did, "It was humiliating in a way. It's like, how can this be? I'm mature now, I'm a grown-up, I'm ready to come into myself, and now I can't sit in the meeting without turning beet red." Both responses offer information, but they lead to dramatically different levels of understanding about menopause and about the look and feel of adequate care and support.

> "I feel like there should be a whole, 'Hey, you're forty, these are some things that are coming up, and here's our health services division for you.' All the women's health services are focused on the baby apparatus, and once you're not making babies or you're not going to have a baby, everything else is a little bit hand-wavy, you know?"—JENNIFER

IS MENOPAUSE A BIG DEAL?

Allopathic medicine has made incredible advances in addressing and treating acute diseases and traumatic injuries. Though there has been progress, managing or preventing chronic and systemic conditions like heart disease, mental illness, endometriosis, and menopause has proved more difficult. The structure of modern medicine separates the systems and areas of the body into its component parts, which become distinct focuses of study. Most practitioners in this system become experts in one specific area or system of the body such as cardiology, ophthalmology, or gynecology. Specialists are trained to isolate conditions by their discrete, ideally microscopic, causes rather than to look more broadly or systemically. Practitioners of alternative medicine systems such as Traditional Chinese Medicine and naturopathic medicine are trained to take a more holistic view of patients, which means they treat the whole body, not just the problem areas. There are exceptions to specialization in modern medical training—general practitioners, family doctors—but these practitioners often refer patients to specialists whenever care that goes beyond preventative measures may be necessary.

Many of the common experiences of the menopause transition—headaches, heart palpitations, disrupted sleep, depression, weight gain, and low libido—can be caused by a variety of things, namely genetics, stress, lifestyle, environment, and dysfunction in another system of the body. The interconnectedness of our body's systems can make it challenging to declare fluctuating sex hormones the definitive culprit. Even though hormones are central to the menopause transition, even endocrinologists consider menopause to be a matter of the reproductive system. Recent research has shown that menopause is also a major neurological transition, but you'd be hard pressed to find a neurologist willing to discuss hot flashes or vaginal dryness with you.

One might imagine that doctors specializing in women's health—obstetricians and gynecologists—would provide education about menopause to patients in their mid to late thirties, but they don't. These specialists are largely focused on fertility, pregnancy, and disease, which are all incredibly important parts of sexual health. Unfortunately, the widespread nature of menopause, with hormonal shifts that prompt recalibration within nearly every system in the body, makes it the purview of everyone in the medical profession, not just within one specialty. Stephanie Faubion, medical director of the North American Menopause Society, referred to the "menopause management vacuum" in an interview with the *New York Times* in 2021: "Until internists and family medicine doctors see menopause as a threat to health in general, they're not going to take it seriously. They're going to say, 'This is one of those female things that will go away.'"

In addition, most medical schools don't provide much menopause education. The North American Menopause Society has made some attempt to fill this gap by offering a Menopause Specialist certification and publishing a clinician's guide to menopause. The fact that menopause is a bit of a hot potato among modern medicine practitioners makes it hard for those going through it to understand who to talk to about what, and whether or not it's a big deal. Unlike puberty, which, at minimum, is covered in health education at school, and pregnancy, which everyone from doctors to overbearing family members is happy to discuss, menopause often does not come up in clinical or personal conversations until it's underway.

"My ex-mother-in-law (she's like ninety-nine now or something), she said, 'They'll tell you headaches have nothing to do with menopause.' It's ridiculous because doctors, at least back in my day, had a pretty narrow set of things that they associated with menopause and a certain time frame that all that was supposed to fit in, and if you started talking about stuff that didn't fit in it, they just dismissed it." —DEANNE

Once menopause conversations start happening there are additional hurdles to clear. Both practitioners and patients are often frustrated about the limited time they have for each appointment—a constraint within our current healthcare and insurance systems. The nuance and depth needed for a thorough discussion about changes in sexual desire or mental health concerns are hard to swing inside a twelve-minute appointment window, especially when the people involved meet infrequently (sometimes only once a year) and one of them is typing notes into a computer. Even if you have the resources to access alternative practitioners with longer appointment times, the information you receive from practitioners can be rife with mixed messages. *What your body is doing is normal. Your body is responding poorly to your fluctuating hormones. The transition can begin as early as your mid-thirties. You can't be in perimenopause if you're still having regular periods.* A conflict arises from the friction between the medical understanding of the menopause transition in *the body* and the lived experience you have as it unfolds in *your body.*

Friends, family, and the internet may also offer information that conflicts with what you hear from your medical practitioner. Are those aches in your joints whispers of perimenopause? Is the acne that's taken up residence on your upper thighs being caused by your new leggings instead of changes in your hormones? Newspapers and magazines are littered with stories of women, especially women subject to racial, class, and fat bias, whose concerns about changes and/or pain in their body are disregarded by medical professionals. Some of these stories end with a simple explanation, others with a visit to a new practitioner who listens and offers support, but some end with the dismissed women finding themselves in emergency medical situations. All of this makes it hard to know when and how hard to argue your case.

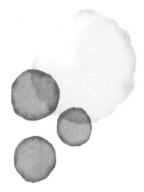

"It's really disorienting, and as a woman and a therapist, it's kind of doubly disorienting because I'm experiencing simultaneously the reality of what's happening on top of being in a culture that says it's like, the end times for your life. Like, hello—I'm walking down this tunnel of hell alone and I'm still expected to function at the same levels inside of this? It's just, sad, you know." —SARA

THE MENOPAUSE THE MARKET IS SELLING

It's wonderful that we are reconsidering the idea of menopause as a physiological cliff in our development. Unfortunately, the physical changes that come with the menopause transition—loosening or folding of the skin, thinning or graying hair, a drier vagina—are not always welcomed by society with open arms. Activist Sonya Renee Taylor does not mince words when describing the mechanics (and intentions) at play in modern capitalism in her book *The Body Is Not an Apology*: "Global capitalism profits from our body shame. . . .

Profit-greedy industries work with media outlets to offer us a distorted perception of ourselves and then use that distorted self-image to sell us remedies for the distortion."

Those experiencing disruptive menopause symptoms need both immediate relief and adequate time and support to take care of themselves without suffering economic losses as a result. Unfortunately, slowing down does not align with the nonstop productivity that the market demands, so most menopause products focus on work-arounds that enable us to keep up. Slogans like "Tame your menopause" and "Menopause doesn't stand a chance" effectively blur the line between empowering people to feel good in their bodies and encouraging them to control their bodies by maintaining a specific appearance or level of productivity.

Whether you receive pay for all of them or not, there are likely multiple types of work you have to do in a given day, at your job, in your relationships, and in your family. Anything that gets in the way of fulfilling your duties in those roles is usually perceived as a problem with *you*, or at least a problem that you're expected to solve. Consumer-oriented menopause products are designed to provide relief, but often they're designed to stop (or slow) you from changing. Because we understand the expectations of the world we live in, we ask for these products—the ones that promise to keep us looking "good," sleeping hard, feeling sexy, and thinking clearly. As author Jia Tolentino writes in *Trick Mirror: Reflections on Self-Delusion*, "Resistance to a system is presented on the terms of the system. It's so much easier, when we gain agency, to adapt rather than to oppose."

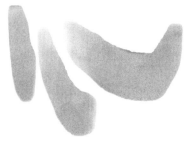

"On average, a woman spends three to five years bleeding. We knew that a process was going to come; we lived our lives around [it], making sure we have the right materials to deal with it, being bummed out when we bled in Starbucks, and years of knowing this egg would come and it would shed, and that had a currency—if your body could do that. Then it's just not there anymore, and your body suddenly is not useful anymore; the means of production is over, so you are too."—SARA

Sometimes it's easy to tell when a company or product is preying on your concerns—teeth-whitening kits and wrinkle cream come to mind—but other times it's tricky to discern whether something you're experiencing is a problem or something you've been led to *believe* is a problem. On matters of your appearance, the answer may be both: you might not mind gray hair personally and also be aware that it could work against you in the job market. There is also a real possibility that the changes you experience in your body and mind during menopause will arrive before you feel ready for them.

Regardless of where the pressure originates from, it can inspire you to rebel in the form of expensive anti-aging serum, a younger lover, Botox, higher hemlines, or "boot camp" workouts. In our youth-obsessed culture, these products and behaviors are at once perpetuating a negative narrative about aging and responding to a valid set of concerns given the cultural context we live in. There are consequences to not adhering to the script. In *Belabored: A Vindication of the Rights of Pregnant Women*, Lyz Lenz articulates the central message of the script succinctly: "The advice was still—as always—control yourself, woman."

The market for menopause products and services has been called a "gold rush" by journalists; perimenopause alone is an estimated ten-billion-dollar market that grows by 6,000 new "customers" every day in the United States alone. You are a target in this expanding market, but also this is not your first rodeo. There is no universally right way to move through this experience as a consumer, because each individual comes into it with a unique combination of needs. Trust your gut, your bullshit detector, and—let's not forget—your hackles to help you navigate a path that suits you, and support others by giving them space to do the same, even when they make choices that are different from yours.

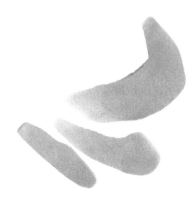

CULTURE: THE MENOPAUSE YOU'VE HEARD ABOUT

Every minute of your life is lived in your body. All your experiences are mediated through your body and also influenced by the ways others perceive and assign value to it. There are messages about menopause floating around in movies, jokes, chat rooms, and the stories you hear from or about people in the midst of it. These public perceptions color your experiences, even if only because of the effort it requires to resist them. Cultural tropes about menopause and aging are intertwined— wrinkling skin, fat accumulating around midsections, dried-up vaginas, misery, and shrill tones—and unified by the theme of bodies and behaviors becoming increasingly problematic as we progress through life.

Your body is like a set of hangers for an entire wardrobe of cultural ideas, perceptions, and assumptions. Some of them were designed in collaboration with you, or at the very least were chosen by you, but many were selected by other people or institutions. We are generally aware of the ways, imagined and real, that other people see and don't see us. Whether it's a matter of experiencing hot flashes in the workplace (public) or explaining to a new sexual partner (private) that penetrative sex or touch is currently uncomfortable, both changes in your body are made visible to other people.

We all have expectations about our bodies that are formed by our environment—cultural, geographical, familial—and those expectations are constantly being reinforced or challenged as we move through different physiological experiences—injuries, pregnancy, growth spurts, aging—and as we move through spaces where we look more or less like the people around us. We are generally prepared to navigate certain kinds of friction, like the kind that arises when others respond to a dramatic change in our clothing or hairstyle, but less prepared for being seen through transitions that feel beyond our control or that we know are culturally contentious. Like all other physiological experiences from birth through death, menopause is a transition within your body that is swaddled in a quilt of cultural meaning.

"It would be nice if there was some threshold ritual that women experienced when they were going through menopause. Everyone makes fun of men when they're going through the midlife crisis because they buy a fancy car and get a younger girlfriend; I would even like to see that in the culture: *Oh she's going through menopause, yeah now she's like polyamorous and a cougar or whatever.*" —MAUDE

Like your identity, your cultural home is not a singular dwelling. It is more like the Winchester Mystery House: an eclectic smattering of rooms, additions, closets, and flourishes that are assembled from your relationships, circumstances, and choices. The larger culture that we inhabit together is experienced differently by each of us, and sometimes it can be hard to discern your actual experience from what you've been told to expect. Unpacking and examining the cultural narratives surrounding menopause is a way to remind ourselves that these stories are merely ideas that were built and reinforced over time rather than truths that dictate our experience. The following stereotypes are just a few that I hear and see most persistently (which does not make them true). My hope is that starting a conversation about this topic will make the constructs visible, allowing us to begin the work of dismantling them and reminding us that we can build new ones.

MENOPAUSE IS THE GATEWAY TO OLD

Menopause represents the end of not one but two intertwined and deeply treasured facets of the female identity in our culture: youth and fertility. It's not surprising that we don't like to think, let alone talk, about it. Tropes of raging, red-faced middle-aged women perpetuate the assumption that everyone going through menopause is middle-aged. Although the majority of people who will experience menopause will do so in their middle years, there are others who go through this transition at other chronological ages as a result of their genetics, health history, or other lived experiences. A cursory review of content aimed at menopausal people confirms that not only is middle age when people are beginning to look and feel old but also that looking or feeling old is a problem that can and should be addressed.

Age can feel like a sneaker wave, a force that arrives without warning and with surprising impact. You might experience it physically, realizing one day that an activity you've done a million times is much more challenging than it used to be or now comes with harsh consequences, or emotionally, feeling bewildered when a group of your coworkers wishes you a happy thirty-fifth birthday with a wink and a smile even though they all know that you're turning forty-five (true story!).

In her book *This Chair Rocks: A Manifesto against Ageism,* ageism activist Ashton Applewhite makes a powerful distinction: "Fear of dying is human, fear of aging is cultural." If you are resistant to aging, your position is not without good reason. We are taught in subtle and overt ways to treasure youth and dread aging. Midlife and menopause are part of growing older. We are not short on negative associations with aging—slow, sick, lonely, asexual, reliant—and as a result old age is not a place many of us are looking forward to. It's not difficult to understand how a person going through menopause would resist or at least begrudge being categorized as an aging person, nor is it a stretch to see how those going through it earlier than anticipated might struggle to make sense of the transition or to locate themselves in public menopause constructs and conversations.

Applewhite employs cold, hard logic to our attitudes about aging, asking why we celebrate change and growth until midlife and then do the opposite. I appreciate her inquiry, and I can also see how, in my own life, the changes and growth I imagined in my twenties and thirties were about accruing experiences, knowledge, relationships, and skills; things looked possible because I felt like I had plenty of time. The changes I imagine in my later years are centered around a decrease in the pace of growth or in access to opportunities—in other words, loss. My belief that the aperture of possibilities in my own life is narrowing can make things feel paradoxically pointless and urgent. I can't be sure whether the possibilities are truly dwindling or if it's only that my imagination around aging is a bit anemic. How might menopause look different if we could imagine an affirmative view of aging?

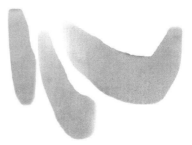

"Before I was going through this, the thought of going through the stage, that's like to be put up on a shelf, to be put away, like you're winding down. . . . In truth, you're not winding down. You have some years left, and the people that have been demanding your time aren't going to necessarily demand anymore—like divorce or kids growing up. But it's not like, *Oh, that poor person,* it's like, *Yay, that person!* Hopefully they have a good relationship with all those people, and they can all go and do other things. I feel like there's a sad thing of, *Oh, that poor lady,* and that's what I'm shying away from—that part of menopause. Don't feel sorry for me, even though I do need tenderness right now."

— SHEILA

Heather Corrina, educator and activist, wrote in her recent book *What Fresh Hell Is This? Perimenopause, Menopause, Other Indignities, and You* about the tension that comes with big transitions and how the feelings you have about them depend greatly on what it is you believe you are transitioning to. Ageism is thriving in Western culture; the tether between menopause and aging can create a shift in identity that you don't feel ready to embody. Many of us have had the experience of reaching an anticipated age (often the "big" ones like eighteen, forty, seventy) only to find that the way you feel at that age doesn't align with what you imagined. That disconnect is an opening, a scrap of evidence that aging, old, and older are less defined territories than we think.

"I mean, it is fundamentally, for most people, going to be harder to go through this transition than the one from child to maiden because we're getting closer to death, you know, and also we're going to have less energy. And energy is nice. We want to contribute, we want to be around for others, and that actually takes a little bit of energy." —MAUDE

MENOPAUSE IS A WHITE LADY THING

Physiologically speaking, all people with ovaries will go through one of the types of menopause outlined in chapter 1. However, given the emphasis on white women as representations of the feminine in everything from fashion to pharmaceuticals, it's easy to see how BIPOC individuals wouldn't see themselves in modern menopause as it is represented in popular culture or advertisements. Data collected in the SWAN study suggests that menopause unfolds differently among racial and ethnic groups of women in terms of timing, duration, and specific symptoms experienced. For example, Black women report more hot flashes and night sweats, and Hispanic women more often report vaginal and urogenital symptoms, like dryness and leaking. Research also shows that race and class affect how menopause is perceived, the kind of care or support people seek, and the level of care they receive.

"This thing of femaleness and the beautification coming through a white lens . . . looking at pad commercials where she's skipping through the lilies and her hair is flowing, and there's daisies and sunflowers. That was not my earliest experiences with my cycle. And I can appreciate that, of course, that image was there to sell that pad, right? It wasn't to help women to celebrate that space in life, but it's also an image that was connected with the cycle. If your cycle doesn't look like this, especially if you're a Black woman and your cycle doesn't look like this, now you've got a deficit model of having a period. And if you don't have the space where you can define it for yourself, you'll start thinking *something's wrong with me because my period doesn't look like that or feel like that.*" —ALATHEA

The experience of menopause is influenced by all aspects of an individual's identity. Writers, activists, and scholars have documented the unique and varied concerns women of color have historically brought to their organizing work, including their work around reproductive rights and freedoms. Black, Asian Pacific Islander, Latinx, and Indigenous feminists all came to the reproductive health conversation with an understanding that ethnic identity affects women's mental and physical health through policies on everything from immigration to the environment, through economics, and through social structures that create and reinforce class, race, and gender oppression. Menopause will likely continue to look like a white lady thing until our country makes significant strides toward more equitable access to resources including wealth, opportunity, and healthcare.

Oh, and It's Cisgender and Heterosexual Too!

Every aspect of women's reproductive health—puberty, pregnancy, menopause—that is culturally shared is often presented through the dominant narrative: cisgender, heterosexual, and often white. Other narratives are emerging, but it's going to take time to evolve our cultural understanding of the full range of identities that people going through menopause can embody.

Look no further than the ways that symptoms of menopause like depression or mood swings were marketed as marital problems throughout the twentieth century. Therapist and queer menopause researcher Tania Glyde has articulated the unique challenges a queer person can face in their transition to menopause as a direct result of menopause being persistently presented as a cisgender, heteronormative experience. If a queer person is challenged by their perimenopause symptoms, there could be an additional layer of concern that their struggle will be viewed as normative. Concerns about that perception might prevent a queer person from seeking or accepting the help that they need.

MENOPAUSE IS A CLOAK OF INVISIBILITY

I remember how hot my face flushed the day that I stood in the coffee shop down the street from my apartment and waited for the person at the register to notice me, the sole customer waiting to place an order. He looked up and then what felt like right through me, to the shelves of merchandise on the wall behind me, before beginning to restock the pastry case. After a couple of minutes that felt like more like twenty, I walked out. I think of myself as the kind of person who speaks up, but that barista's vacant stare did me in. I scurried home and wondered if something about my presence or presentation had rendered me unworthy of notice. I have no idea what actually happened that day in the cafe, but I know how quickly and effortlessly I dropped into the narrative: something about the way I looked made me unworthy of being noticed in public.

It's one thing to be overlooked when you're trying to order a coffee, but people in the midst of menopause also talk about having this experience in terms of diminished power in their jobs, communities, and relationships. It isn't necessarily an underlying desire to be perceived as sexy, but instead an awareness that being noticed in that way is a form of power, a means of commanding attention. Not all people who go through menopause will experience a dramatic shift in their sense of being visible to people typically in power in our society: cisgender, heterosexual, white men. For some, feeling a sense of invisibility within the structures of power will not be a new experience.

Attention based on physical appearance is a double-edged sword, both for women and for those with identities that don't fit into the culturally constructed gender binary. When the subject of attention from men arose in my conversations with women, people generally expressed a sense of relief that they no longer had to contend with *unwanted* attention. While my interviewees did not express sadness around this loss, I have heard (and read) women describe missing and even grieving the decline in the sexual attention they attract. It's hard not to feel self-conscious or somehow diminished when some form of attention or even consideration that was given or extended to you seems to suddenly disappear.

This feeling of invisibility can follow you around, hovering like a cloud when you're with family, at the doctor's office, or out clothes shopping, partly because midlife feels ambiguous: it's neither the beginning nor the end of something. The culturally entrenched markers of adulthood like college, marriage, children, and homeownership have either been checked off or not, and there is scant definition, besides the marker of death at the end, for the time that lies ahead of you. It's as confusing for the people you interact with as it is for you because there is no obvious hook for a conversation, no central theme of your life around which your interaction can orbit. People don't know what they are seeing when they see you, and it's possible that you don't either.

"When I was growing up, in literature and film the only older women that ever had any agency or power were witches and fairy-tale queens. There's a sense of purposelessness to it; even if you still work, even if you still have kids, there's a strain. Like you might still have these roles—I'm a teacher, or I'm a writer, or I'm a mother—but the closer you get to retirement and children leaving, what are you then?" —MAUDE

Some people experience this amoebic identity as freedom, loving the way it allows them to shape-shift, slipping in between and among identities. Others are flooded with a sense of uncertainty or destabilized by their shifting status in social and professional circles. There are forces at play that are beyond your control here, but you also have a say about how you inhabit yourself, regardless of whether and how you are seen.

"The perimenopausal period, it's also a period in women's lives when, for many of us, life can be pretty stressful. You might be in a marriage and raising kids and marriages are hard and raising kids is hard and you have a job and marriage is not all it's cracked up to be. So that irritability or depression or flashes of anger, well, is that because something is changing in my body or is that because I'm just pissed off because the forties is really a hard decade?"—DEANNE

PART TWO

|

What Could It Be Like for You?

3

ALL THAT COULD HAPPEN FROM PERI- TO POSTMENOPAUSE

Most of us learned about our reproductive system either in health class, from an awkward conversation with a parent or guardian, or via found reference material—online or analog. The information was probably presented in the context of sexual activity, mainly the potential for pregnancy and contracting sexually transmitted diseases. Focusing so tightly on sex and reproduction itself, we don't learn about the connection between our menstrual cycle and our overall health, which can make the widespread bodily changes during the transition to menopause—like brain fog and joint pain—confounding. How could changes in the hormones that run my ovaries do that?

We tend to think that menopause only involves our reproductive system, when in reality the shifts in our sex hormone levels impact our whole body because estrogen and progesterone have receptors far beyond your pelvic bowl. Your neurological, cardiovascular, endocrine, musculoskeletal, digestive, and vision systems and your skin have to recalibrate to changing sex hormone levels during and after your menopause transition. Some of the impacts of the menopause transition have a higher probability of being temporary (brain fog, hot flashes), while others are either the beginning or an indicator of longer arcs of change in your health trajectory (such as vaginal dryness and increased risk of cardiovascular disease).

Most doctors and researchers are aware of the reach of your sex hormones and the resulting broad impacts of menopause, but they still do not understand all the mechanics. Even if you don't learn what your sex hormones are doing at every one of their receptor sites throughout your body, it's still useful to know where those receptor sites are located, because your first symptom could be outside of your reproductive system. You might experience changes to your mood, sleep, or cognition long before your menstrual cycle shifts. There is a widespread (and incorrect) perception that the first symptom of perimenopause is a change in the menstrual cycle—longer, shorter, heavier, or lighter—and this can lead people, medical professionals included, to miss other signs of perimenopause or attribute them to another cause.

Every menopause book includes a list of the symptoms that are most frequently reported by people during their transitions to menopause. Please remember that this or any other list of symptoms does not paint a picture of perimenopause as experienced by any singular person. It's more like a visual representation of multiverse theory, where all possible futures are layered onto a single canvas. *You could experience a few, a couple, or none of these symptoms, and you won't know which it will be until you get there.*

"At first, I was just getting all acne all over. Some of my friends were mid-forties and some of them are getting chubbier—like my best friend is getting chubbier—and I'm getting skinnier and bonier, and then I was getting all this acne and maybe more hair. I called my friend and I said, 'I feel I'm turning into a man; I have all this energy.'" —SHEILA

If there's no way to know which symptoms you will experience nor tips for avoiding them, why bring them up? Great question. Because perimenopause is different for everyone, a list of the most commonly reported symptoms is a means of describing what the perimenopause experience *might* entail. Being aware of the ways—physiological and emotional—that shifting hormone levels can manifest as symptoms can help you manage fear and stress and prompt you to seek support early on and advocate for yourself to obtain the care you need and want.

Before you dive into this list, remind yourself that *any symptoms you do experience during your transition to menopause are not your fault.* In the absence of education and discussion about potential perimenopause symptoms, we often find other ways—personal failing is a very popular one—to explain the changes we observe in ourselves. There is a pervasive idea in our culture that it is possible to keep your body—weight, mood, skin—under control if you live the "right way" and follow all the rules. The suggestion that our bodies are controllable may sound empowering, but in truth it shunts blame on those whose bodies do not align with ideals that were constructed centuries ago (and that are continually reinforced by a capitalist system that profits off our vulnerabilities). As Ashton Applewhite deftly articulates in her book *This Chair Rocks*, dissatisfaction can be monetized, self-acceptance cannot.

Is Menopause Part of Aging?

In addition to chronological age, genetics and lived experiences help determine your physiological aging trajectory. Early signs of aging often arise concurrently with perimenopause for those who begin their menopause transition in their mid to late forties. Unless you are going through early menopause, many of the symptoms described here, like skin and body composition changes, can be at least partially attributed to age.

I've read several articles and books authored by people who insist that menopause is not aging, and I can't help but see their assertiveness on this point as an understandably defensive stance in a culture where aging has overwhelmingly negative connotations.

Visible signs of aging in the body don't align with the same chronological ages for everyone, nor do they inform our felt age. Researchers do make distinctions between chronological age and felt age. Research studies that reflect people's thoughts and sentiments pre- and postmenopause show that premenopausal people believe that menopause will make them feel old, but postmenopausal people do not consistently feel old.

Whenever something changes in my body—like when I started having recurring bouts of vertigo—I want to know two things: why is it happening, and how do I fix it? If you are experiencing unfamiliar and potentially unpleasant symptoms, these questions are likely also on your mind. The matter of why perimenopause symptoms happen seems straightforward, and yet even that is challenging to generalize about. This is in part because more research is needed and also because each of us is the medical equivalent of a snowflake—similar in many ways, but also different.

And as for fixing things, this is even trickier because menopause is a *change*, not a brokenness. While there are many treatment options that can manage, and often lessen, the impact of disruptive symptoms, it's not possible, nor is it the goal of researchers or practitioners, to stop menopause from happening. If there is part of you that wants to put this book down and search for a book or magazine article that will tell you that you can take a pass on menopause, I get it. Menopause is a tug at the sleeve from your body, reminding you that you don't call all the shots. It is challenging to accept that you do not have total control over your body—influence, yes; control, no—and it also means you can stop beating yourself up for that long list of things you think could be better if only you had made different choices.

We won't get into the details about tools for managing symptoms (pharmaceuticals, supplements, lifestyle, etc.) here. (We will cover that in part three, along with a variety of things you might consider to help set yourself up for a steadier go through your transition.) Right now, we're going to learn how these symptoms can feel in your body and your life, what scientists know about what causes them, and how to know when it's wise to seek a professional opinion about what's going on in your body. Know that, if you experience some of these symptoms, they might not feel exactly how I've described them here. As a writer I know that words not only matter, they can also mean slightly different things to each of us. Anywhere you see the word *practitioner* it represents whichever type of medical professional you currently have access to—and hopefully feel comfortable with—for your healthcare needs.

When Should I Definitely Contact a Medical Professional?

If reading through this lengthy list of potential symptoms is too much right now, that's okay. But there are a few that I want to bring to your attention because, though they can be benign, they can also be signs of more serious health issues. All the symptoms listed here can be caused by perimenopause, other health issues, or both. In the description of each symptom there are indicators for how to gauge what's "normal" versus "a problem," but *these five symptoms always warrant a conversation with, if not a visit to, your practitioner.*

1. **HEART PALPITATIONS:** Yes, these could be perimenopause-related. *And*, it's your heart. Don't mess.

2. **ABNORMAL BLEEDING:** Not only can this disrupt your daily life, it can be caused by many things besides perimenopause—some simple, some not so simply or friendly—so it's good practice to check it out.

3. **FATIGUE:** Everyone is tired a lot of the time, but intense fatigue that renders you unable to participate in day-to-day life warrants investigation. Same goes for joint pain.

4. **VULVOVAGINAL ITCHING:** Maybe this is part of your perimenopause experience, but there are half a dozen other causes for it too. Menopause related or not, many of these will get worse without treatment.

5. **POSTMENOPAUSAL BLEEDING:** Anything from a blob to a tiny spot should be reported and checked out. This can be serious, even uterine precancer or uterine cancer.

BODY SHAPE AND SIZE CHANGES

One week you're putting your clothes on in the morning just like everybody else, and the next week everything fits differently or straight up does not fit at all. Almost everyone has experienced a change in their body shape at some point during their life, but for those who experience the menopause transition during midlife, these changes can be confounding because they seem to materialize from the ether. Changes in body composition are common throughout peri- and postmenopause and tend to rank high on the list of symptoms that come with significant emotional impact.

During midlife, age- and hormone-related changes make bodily systems and processes like metabolism work differently, and that affects the amount (more) and location (your middle) of fat stored and how much (less) lean muscle mass you have. These changes can throw you for a loop because you're just living your life, doing stuff the same way you always have, and all of a sudden not one of your

WHAT COULD IT BE LIKE FOR YOU?

pairs of pants fits. The reality of midlife is that your routines, habits, and behaviors have new and different consequences than they did in the past because of naturally occurring changes in metabolism and muscle development.

Fat accumulated during this time tends to cluster around the midsection. This abdominal fat is sometimes called adipose fat and has been shown to increase risk of heart disease and diabetes. Aerobic exercise and strength training become increasingly important as you move into midlife, not so much to guarantee that you'll continue to wear the same-size clothes, but to help you maintain or even rebuild lean muscle mass and to keep abdominal fat in check. The goal is to ensure that you're able to do the activities you need and want to do for as long as possible.

Unfortunately, messaging from the weight loss and weight management industry focuses our attention on adhering to a narrow, fixed aesthetic standard rather than a functional one that evolves over the course of our lives. The notion of the ideal female form is deeply rooted in patriarchal ideology that defines beautiful as white, thin, and young. When our bodies do not conform to this standard, they are considered unruly, and by association, we are considered irresponsible. Global capitalism has profited immensely off our insecurities and shame by selling us age-defying lotions, fat-flattening panties, and anti-calorie cleanses. These products tell us in no uncertain terms that we should always be striving for the "ideal" form.

The medical establishment has not helped matters by codifying beliefs that all bodies should be held to a single standard, that we all should be close to the same weight. Body mass index (BMI) is a measurement that medical professionals use as a tool in assessing overall health. Earlier we discussed the risks inherent in the notion of a norm or standard for all bodies, and BMI has come under scrutiny in recent decades because it asserts that there is a healthy weight-to-height ratio, that is true for all bodies.

Weight management and nutrition compose one of the most confusing corners of the medical field and are an unmitigated disaster on the internet. It is not possible, or logical, for me to position any conversation about weight as strictly a matter of health, because science and medicine are practiced by people who can (and do) discriminate against bodies that do not conform to the long-established standard that says thin is healthy. Considering our culture's fixation on thinness, it's not surprising that scientific research confirms a marked bias among health professionals against higher weight bodies. Experts are only just beginning to look at how this kind of bias might also be contributing to differences in care and, ultimately, in patient outcomes.

The Health at Every Size movement explores the possibility that bodies can regulate themselves at a wider variety of weights than we've historically considered acceptable. More research is needed, but there are studies that have shown that changes in behavior— stress reduction, increased movement—can influence health outcomes as much as, if not more than, weight loss. It's important to note that Health at Every Size is not a rallying cry for disregarding body fat amounts and distribution as risk factors for diabetes, cardiovascular disease, or cancer. It is a reasoned argument to more carefully examine the exact relationship between body size and health outcomes.

CAUSES

Some doctors refer to midlife as the perfect storm for changes to body shape and composition. The demands of midlife—work and financial pressure, shifting family and relationship dynamics, changes in health—can leave us feeling depleted but also keep us from being nourished and rested. It may be more difficult to exercise for a variety of reasons including limited energy, time, or resources, and potentially even a lack of safety at the time of day you could feasibly fit in some movement. These pressures are real, and as a result, most of us will become more sedentary as we age.

Your metabolism naturally slows down as a result of aging, making it easier to gain weight even when you're eating and moving exactly the same way that you have for years. Muscle mass also declines with age, which affects your strength and tips your lean muscle to fat ratio in favor of fat. There is an uptick in muscle mass decline during the menopause transition, which means that the amount of energy required by your muscles also declines and your body doesn't need the same number of calories that it used to. At the same time, age and hormone-related changes in the body lead to an increased potential for insulin resistance. Let's take a closer look at this.

"Even when I've carried this much weight on my body in the past, I never had a paunchy lower abdomen. It's probably the most painful part of all of this, because I was so vain about my flat stomach, and musculature that resembled maybe a four-pack. And right now, I can't find my stomach anymore. When I look down at the waistband of my jeans, I just see a giant fat-baby, and someone else's body." —NICOLE

Metabolism is the name for the process where your body converts what you eat and drink into energy it can use. Your body wants to maintain a steady supply of fuel—not too much, not too little—to keep all your cells fed and functioning. When you eat and drink, your blood sugar (aka glucose) levels naturally rise. In response to more glucose in your blood, your pancreas releases a hormone called insulin that ferries glucose around your body and makes it available to your cells. When glucose levels are elevated, your body stores any excess glucose in your liver as glycogen, a storable form of glucose that can be released back into the bloodstream as glucose at some point in the future when blood sugar is low.

Metabolism works best when blood sugar fluctuates gently rather than in the abrupt spikes and drops that the refined-carbohydrate-rich Western diet is known to create. Processed foods, fried foods, sweets, and starchy things make your blood sugar levels jump up and your pancreas pump out insulin to move as much sugar as possible, as quickly as possible, to your cells. When that influx of sugar drops off, you experience the feeling of a crash in your energy that makes you crave more carbs and sugar. When we chronically produce too much insulin in response to a lot of glucose in our blood, our body loses the ability to keep up, and we end up with both high sugar and high insulin. Eventually, our pancreas and its insulin response cannot adapt to this high-stakes process, resulting in type 2 diabetes, which creates a burden on our body's systems and organs.

Insulin resistance describes what happens when cells no longer respond to insulin. They ignore the request from insulin to accept glucose, and the brain and cells throughout the body can end up being starved for energy as a result. Relentless sugar cravings can sometimes be the result of chronically low blood sugar caused by insulin resistance rather than a willpower problem. When insulin and blood sugar are dysregulated from the day before, you don't wake up in the best state, and this prompts you to repeat the cycle of peaking and crashing for days, weeks, or potentially years. When you become insulin resistant, your blood sugar levels stay elevated and you store fat more easily. It also negatively impacts muscle mass, because one of insulin's roles is promoting muscle development.

Researchers are still debating whether insulin resistance leads to weight gain or weight gain causes insulin resistance, but they do know that both of these conditions make us more likely to develop type 2 diabetes. Research on sex differences and insulin resistance suggests that estrogen plays a protective role, helping pre-menopausal people to maintain insulin sensitivity. As estrogen declines through the menopause transition, some of that protection is lost.

WHEN SHOULD I BE CONCERNED?

Many people, though not all, gain weight during menopause and gain weight in new areas of their bodies. The challenges this presents are real, because we've been trained to believe that weight gain is never acceptable. Corporations have leveraged our fears about changes in body shape and size to sell us more products and services. As a result, disordered eating—yo-yo dieting, restricted eating, compulsive eating, and anxiety associated with food, eating, and exercise—has been normalized. In an interview with journalist Anne-Helen Petersen, author and fellow journalist, Virginia Sole-Smith noted how skilled fatphobia's proponents are at dressing a wolf in sheep's clothing: "The food movement became wellness culture, which is just diet culture rebranded by Gwyneth Paltrow."

As challenging as it is to continually discover that your clothes do not fit your new body shape, it is not an indication that something has gone terribly wrong. It is, in fact, a highly predictable outcome. An increase in fat might be bad news for your wardrobe, but it's not necessarily bad news for your health; it all depends on your body composition (and overall health) prior to an increase in fat and, to some degree, where the fat is accumulating.

Measuring your middle will tell you more about your risk profile than stepping on a scale. If you're accumulating fat in your abdominal area (aka adipose fat), that's something you want to discuss with your practitioner, because there is a correlation between increased adipose fat and increased risk of heart disease and diabetes. Food cravings—specifically for carb-heavy and sweet stuff—or feeling light-headed or shaky on a regular basis can be indicators that you are in the peak-and-crash blood sugar cycle that leads to insulin resistance. These are both important things to talk about with your practitioner to understand if there is a way for you to maintain a more stable level of energy and experience satiety, not just fullness, from your meals and snacks.

Movement is good for you physically and emotionally. If you are finding it difficult to continue with the activities that keep you moving, whatever they are, because of physical discomfort or breathlessness, or because of anxiety as a result of the first two,

reach out to your practitioner to discuss. It may be that you need to change up your activity or allow time for healing and recovery. Either way, you want to make sure that you are on a path back to a level of activity that keeps you feeling good and supports your overall health. Note that the path to health does not *always* include weight loss.

COGNITIVE CHANGES: BRAIN FOG, MEMORY LOSS

If all of a sudden you are losing track of things like your phone, house keys, or parked car, you are not alone. Cognitive change complaints including difficulty remembering things and the inability to focus are common throughout the menopause transition. Some people experience a level of cognitive change that makes it a challenge to complete daily tasks at work or keep tabs on things at home.

CAUSES

Fluctuating estrogen levels impact specific regions of the brain associated with various symptoms of perimenopause: the hypothalamus (body temperature regulation), brain stem (sleep/wake cycles), and amygdala/hippocampus (mood swings and forgetfulness). Also remember that other symptoms of menopause— lack of sleep, changes in mood, anxiety, and physical discomfort— can have a negative impact on memory and ability to focus, so this symptom can be a challenging one to tease out and identify as a stand-alone issue.

WHEN SHOULD I BE CONCERNED?

Descartes's statement "I think, therefore I am" gets directly to the heart of why changes to the way we think and retain information can be frightening. Drastic changes like the kind of amnesia that can happen with a traumatic event or injury are easier to notice than a slow but steady increase in forgetfulness or decline in attentiveness. If you are struggling to mentally keep up with your day-to-day activities at work or home, it is worth speaking to your practitioner, because, at a minimum, it might be helpful to do some basic cognitive testing that can serve as a baseline for further examination down the road.

The people around you on a daily basis can also be a helpful source of feedback if you feel like something is changing but you're not sure. Obviously, talking to people in your life about concerns you have about your memory or cognitive capacity is complicated because you might worry them, they might lose confidence in you, or they may be dismissive of your concerns. Discussing your concerns in a supportive environment can help you navigate any fear or anxiety you may be experiencing and get emotional or even clinical support that could alleviate your symptoms.

Many people who experience mild cognitive shifts during their transition notice some improvement when they reach postmenopause. Recent research implies that forgetfulness and fogginess improve slightly as people approach menopause, but more research is needed to understand the influence of the menopause transition on both short- and long-term cognitive changes.

> **"There is this feeling that you'll never get [your mind] back. You feel broken, [but] that doesn't last, and women do talk about that. The reassurance around the fact that your brain isn't going to work, or might not work at certain times, is a kindness."**
> **—DEANNE**

JOINT AND MUSCLE PAIN

Chronic musculoskeletal pain can be anywhere in the body but tends to show up in the neck, shoulder, lower back, knees, hands, and hips. As we age, we lose muscle mass and the related connective tissues. People begin to experience the effects of these declines— loss of strength, muscle aches, and stiff joints—in their mid-forties, which can line up with the onset of other perimenopause symptoms. Insomnia, another symptom during the menopause transition, can exacerbate joint and muscle pain and, in some cases, lead to its development.

> "I went to my naturopath and was like, 'What the fuck is this? All of a sudden, out of nowhere, I can't put my arm behind my back. What is this?' And she's like, 'Oh, yeah, we call that menopause shoulder.' I'm like, 'Jesus, why is nobody talking about this? You're telling me that I'm not going to be able to move my joint for, you know, twelve, sixteen, eighteen months, and my option is to get a cortisone shot or not?'" —AIMEE

CAUSES

Researchers aren't certain why, but joint and muscle aches are more common in women than men, and the data points to an uptick in joint and muscle pain in women aged forty-five to fifty-five. No study has made a direct link between estrogen fluctuation or decline and joint

> "I noticed when I exercise, I need downtime or else I'll hurt the next day. My body's not springing back. I love exercise, I'm really physical, and I remember the first time it happened, I did Pilates in the morning and then I wasn't ready for my day like I always am. I felt really horrible, and I was like, *Oh, I need to relax and stretch after Pilates. I can't bounce from thing to thing to thing.*" —Maude

and muscle pain, so most of this discomfort is attributed to a natural, age-related decline in muscle mass and connective tissue. There is some evidence that estrogen plays a role in maintaining healthy connective tissues—cartilage, synovial membranes, ligaments—as well as in joint-adjacent bones and muscles. As hormones decline, connective tissue in your joints becomes less effective, potentially leading to inflammation. Both estrogen and progesterone do have anti-inflammatory effects, and it is possible that the decline of both hormones reduces the body's ability to respond to sustained inflammation as a result of damaged tissue.

WHEN SHOULD I BE CONCERNED?

If your pain is continuously increasing without any relief or is preventing you from participating in your regular daily activities, reach out to your practitioner to discuss.

MENSTRUAL CYCLE CHANGES

"It was a shift in cycle, but mostly elongated, but not by a long, long time, but to the point where—because I was married at the time—I was like, *Shit, am I pregnant?*" —AIMEE

The initial changes to most people's cycles look like cycles getting shorter and bleeding getting heavier. Not everyone will have their cycles get shorter or bleed more (or notice that they do). The first change to hit your radar could be a skipped period or a very late one, which also happens during perimenopause. Some people will not notice any difference in their cycle length or bleeding because they are taking hormonal birth control, which blocks ovulation and can, depending on the formulation, prompt a withdrawal bleed (which is different from a period bleed) on a regular schedule. Considering that the absence of a period for one full year is the marker of arrival at menopause, it can be tricky for those on hormonal birth control to know when they become menopausal.

Some people report that the PMS symptoms they haven't experienced in decades come back or that the ones they always had become worse during their menopause transition. Many will get adequate relief from this discomfort with ibuprofen for two to three days before their period. Some will find that the level of pain they experience increases in intensity or starts happening throughout their cycle.

> "From about age forty-eight to forty-nine, my period happened every 21 to 24 days and lasted between 7 to 10 days each time. Every period had at least two days of—I'll be blunt—like mass murder days where it's just like, *What is happening here?!* I'm not a huge fan of period sex either, so that was another really negative effect for me." —CHELSEA

What Constitutes a "Heavy" Menstrual Flow?

Heavy menstrual flow is a loss of more than 80 ml during one period or bleeding for more than seven days. When you read that up to 80 ml of menstrual fluid is okay, you might roll your eyes and wonder who has ever measured what comes out? You're right, most of us have not, but it is possible to do it with some basic understanding of tampon and menstrual pad absorbency and menstrual cup capacity. If you have a predictable monthly flow, it might be useful to pay attention for one or two cycles and jot down your current menstrual flow amount as a baseline for comparison once you begin to notice changes. If your cycles have always fluctuated considerably, it might still be helpful to track your totals to see if any predictable patterns or unexpected changes emerge.

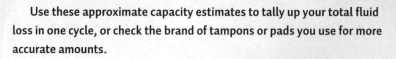

Use these approximate capacity estimates to tally up your total fluid loss in one cycle, or check the brand of tampons or pads you use for more accurate amounts.

1. Fully soaked regular tampon: 5 ml

2. Fully soaked regular menstrual pad: 5 ml

3. Fully soaked super tampon: 10 ml

4. Menstrual cups indicate their capacity; base your calculation on the fullness of the cup

If measuring by fluid volume just does not compute, not to worry; there are some other great reference points. If you are going through super tampons or pads in just a couple of hours, need a combination of tampon and pad to get through the night, or pass clots the size of a quarter or larger, it's time to consult a practitioner to make sure you're not becoming anemic (low iron) or experiencing another health issue that's causing heavy bleeding.

CAUSES

Sex hormone levels directly influence your menstrual cycle. When the ovaries are less responsive, the hypothalamus reads that as a need to prompt the pituitary to send out more FSH, which leads to a frenzy of effort to mature follicles. Because the follicle quality has declined, it becomes less and less likely that an egg will be released. The extra effort to develop more follicles means that cycles are faster and burn through more follicles. Without ovulation, there is no ruptured follicle releasing a supply of progesterone. In the absence of progesterone— which usually mitigates the effects of estrogen—estrogen is left to build the thick uterine wall of its dreams; as a result, your flow can be significantly heavier and last longer than what you typically experience.

A lack of progesterone can also mean an uptick in premenstrual discomforts such as breast pain or cramps. As ovarian function slows and estrogen levels decline overall, periods become less frequent and bleeding is lighter until it eventually stops happening at all. In general, heavy bleeding and other menstrual irregularities occur in the early stages of perimenopause, which, in most cases, lasts between one and three years.

WHEN SHOULD I BE CONCERNED?

Practitioners and individuals alike can fall prey to the assumption that abnormal bleeding occurring in people of a certain age is a symptom of perimenopause, whether it is accompanied by other symptoms or not. If accompanied by pain, abnormal bleeding could be adenomyosis (endometrial tissue growing into the wall of the uterus) or endometriosis (endometrial tissue growing on organs outside the uterus), especially if you're also having spotting between your periods and broader pelvic pain. And there is always a possibility that you have multiple health issues happening at the same time that may or may not be related to your menopausal transition. A super heavy or irregular menses that is not due to an underlying condition—uterine fibroids, uterine polyps, ovarian cysts, endometriosis, adenomyosis, thyroid conditions, or uterine cancer—is called dysfunctional uterine bleeding by medical professionals.

If you bleed at all postmenopause—even spotting or slight tinges of blood on the toilet paper—you absolutely want to let your practitioner know or schedule a visit with them. Bleeding postmenopause could be happening because of a polyp on the cervix, thin vaginal tissue that has become quite delicate, or a sign of uterine cancer.

If you begin to experience pain with your menstrual cycle that cannot be relieved with the use of ibuprofen or you are in pain throughout your cycle or during sex, it's probably time to consult a practitioner. Period and menstrual cycle pain have long been considered normal—which is outrageous—but this is no longer the case as researchers learn more about underlying conditions like fibroids and endometriosis that can cause significant discomfort.

MIGRAINES

Migraines are usually distinct from headaches in that they are often worse on one side of the head than the other and involve a throbbing or pulsating pain. Sensitivity to light or sound, nausea, and vomiting can also be part of a migraine experience. Research shows a connection between headaches and menstruation: 60 percent of women who report migraines say that they are associated with their menstrual cycle in some way. Migraines that come on any time during the two days prior to the onset of menses through the first three days of menses are called *pure menstrual migraines*. Those that happen at other times throughout the menstrual cycle—right when the period is over or maybe right at ovulation—are called *menstrual migraines* because there is a connection to hormonal changes. Most people note that their migraines decrease postmenopause, and those who solely had menstrual migraines say that they often go away completely.

"I used to get really bad hormonal headaches right before my period. Those have not been around for quite some time, and now they are back, but it's harder to identify because I don't have a cycle around them." —AIMEE

WHAT COULD IT BE LIKE FOR YOU?

As we've discussed, hormonal changes become unpredictable and erratic during perimenopause; as a result, people who have these menstrual-related migraines can see them worsen, with greater intensity or frequency. On the other hand, once they're postmenopausal, they will probably have fewer of this type of migraine because estrogen levels aren't fluctuating wildly anymore.

CAUSES

Short answer: Medical professionals don't know for sure. Research data shows that women with a history of migraine headaches of any kind have fewer during pregnancy, and this has led researchers to believe that fluctuating estrogen could play a role in migraines (because estrogen is stable during pregnancy). Progesterone also has receptors in the brain, but its potential role in migraine activity has not been sufficiently studied. Beyond hormonal shifts, other aspects of and influences on brain chemistry and brain physiology can affect the incidence of and one's vulnerability to migraines, including vascular instability, inflammatory cascades, pain receptor glitches, food sensitivities, and genetic and hormonal influences.

WHEN SHOULD I BE CONCERNED?

If you have a history of migraines or other headaches, you'll want to take note if you have a headache of greater intensity or with new symptoms. Whether you are prone to headaches or not, a headache that is accompanied by changes to your speech or vision, cognitive difficulties, or a noticeably elevated level of pain is an indication that it's time to reach out to your practitioner to determine if it warrants further evaluation.

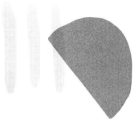

MOOD CHANGES

It's probably not a surprise at this point when I say that perimenopause can affect mood, with results such as depression, anxiety, low motivation, irritability, a short temper, impatience, volatile reactivity, and negative self-talk. The common denominator here is a shift in your experience—some way of responding or reacting or coping that is different from what you were doing before. These changes might remind you of mood changes you've experienced as part of PMS. Of course, anyone can have a bad week or a tough year, but the kinds of mood shifts that are reported during perimenopause are things that leave people saying *I just don't feel like myself*, or *I feel a little unhinged*.

"I cried my way through a work retreat for three days. I was like, *I'm under a lot of stress, and I'm just not coping, and I've got to get it together and bootstrap my way out of this. I'm just having this individual experience. I'm falling apart. I can't get my shit together—what's wrong with me?* It took someone stopping and saying, "Yeah, you probably could get some help with that." My friend told me that with empathy and caring, treating it like something that wasn't about my own fundamental failures." —MELISSA

CAUSES

Although estrogen gets most of the attention in conversations about perimenopause, progesterone levels are also impacted in the early stages of your transition when ovulation happens less reliably. Progesterone has a soothing effect on your nervous system, and without it, or even with significantly less of it, you may notice that your stress level rises or that you experience increased anxiety. Sex hormones have complex interactions with dominant neurotransmitters such as serotonin, dopamine, GABA, and glutamate. Numerous areas of the brain have high densities of estrogen and progesterone receptors, including the amygdala, hypothalamus, and hippocampus. Hormonal transitions such as perimenopause influence neurotransmitters—their levels and transmission—and other brain functions including repair, development, maintenance, and brain structure! When sex hormones shift, neurotransmitters are impacted in ways that affect moods (irritability, anger, depression, anxiety, overwhelm, resilience abilities), cognitive function, and sleep.

As we've discussed, menopause symptoms can be disruptive to your life, and that, in and of itself, may be a source of some irritation or distress. It can be frustrating to spend extra time tending to your body on top of keeping up with the demands of daily life, and that can also affect moods.

> "It's just total volatility, right? Like one minute to the next. My friends call me now, and they're like, 'How are you doing?' I'm like, 'If you had asked me five minutes ago, it would have been really bad and I would have started crying, but right now I'm kind of feeling okay, and that's awesome.' That's today. It's Wednesday. So yeah." —SHEILA

WHEN SHOULD I BE CONCERNED?

Changes to your mood can be easily dismissed as temporary, not that bad, or an isolated incident. They can also be hard to notice in the first place. Sometimes it takes another person checking in and sharing their observations with you for you to see that there is a trend happening or a notable shift in your overall behavior. At the risk of sounding like a robot who penned some mental health content: if you can feel yourself consistently struggling to engage in activities that you normally enjoy, reach out and talk to someone. It sounds rote, and yet it's still a solid measuring device for understanding where you are along the large and nuanced continuum that ranges from deep and unrelenting struggle to thriving. Sometimes it is difficult to observe gradual shifts, especially the internal ones, within yourself. Journaling or even tracking your moods in a rudimentary way—analog or digital—is a helpful tool for noticing changes early on.

Maybe one of your dramatic catchphrases is "I wanted to throw myself in front of a bus" and then one day you realize that you might mean it a little bit. If this is a feeling that you're feeling, don't discredit its power. Talk to someone. Start with people you know, if that has made you feel supported in the past. But if that's not working for any reason, there are other options, like talking to a mental health professional (in person, virtually, or via a crisis hotline). If one-on-one counseling doesn't work for you, locate a support group for people who are experiencing something similar and try that.

Depression or Menopause?

There is considerable overlap in the symptoms of depression and perimenopause: mood changes, disrupted sleep, weight gain, irritability, lack of concentration. But during perimenopause symptoms tend to ebb and flow, whereas a key characteristic of depression is a sustained experience, usually for two weeks or more. It can be helpful to keep tabs on unfamiliar feelings—or familiar feelings that are bigger or more intense than usual— to see if they align with your cycle at all and to note whether they are persistent or intermittent.

Some people are resistant to labeling their symptoms *depression*, at least in part because they fear being prescribed antidepressant medication. This hesitation shows us that there are still stigmas surrounding mental health and broader concerns about treatment options. Although clinical depression is not curable, it is treatable, and medication is not the only option.

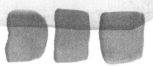

"When I first started noticing that I had more fire and anger, I was like, *Oh, that's really helpful for me* because I've been a pushover a lot of my life and repressed my anger because my mother told me that I should (overtly and covertly) all the time. It was nice to feel like I was channeling this abiding change that all women go through and that we have so many cultural hang-ups about; it felt nice." —MAUDE

SEXUAL CHANGES: INTEREST, DESIRE, DISCOMFORT

One of the biggest myths of menopause is that it crushes the sexual desire of every person who goes through it. This is not consistent with any research that captures what people who have gone through menopause have to say about their interest in sex or satisfaction with the sex they are having. In fact, some report enjoying sex more postmenopause.

There are plenty of words to describe our interest in having sex—libido, randy, sex drive, horny—and these terms have the potential to flatten our experience or relationship to sex into a single dimension: a binary of want it/don't want it. Sexual desire is a nuanced, multifaceted experience, which means that there are many routes to desire and just as many that lead to disinterest or straight-up aversion. Just knowing that a desire for sex or a shift in your sexual satisfaction are menopause symptoms might prompt you to evaluate your sex life more critically. The reality is that, throughout your life, your interest in sex is influenced by a combination of your past experiences and how you feel physically and emotionally in the present.

"I have more libido now than I did in those years. We're freer, and so the response is not as inhibited by either anxiety or the complexity in the relationship, or it can be a more direct experience. When you're younger it's more complicated."

—DEANNE

CAUSES

As I will outline in the discussion of genitourinary syndrome of menopause on page 105, there can be very real changes to tissues in the vagina and pelvic floor that can cause discomfort of pain with sex, especially vaginal penetration. Even without physical discomfort, interest in sex can decline right alongside a decline in overall well-being. Not everyone feels sexy when they're sleep deprived, wrestling with migraines, or anxious that they might sweat through their favorite shirt.

Bona fide changes in hormones, including estrogen levels in women in menopause and testosterone levels in postmenopausal women, are also implicated as causes of lowered desire. Even if everything else is lined up and good to go, these hormonal changes can affect desire and arousal.

There is a very real possibility that decreased sexual desire is *not* caused by something that would be best managed through medical intervention. Even medical reference books like *Clinical Gynecologic Endocrinology and Infertility* say that the two most important influences on sexual interactions of people as they age are the strength of relationships and the physical condition of each partner. Dynamics with your sexual partner(s) and your sexual history with them and others will influence your level of interest in sex. An in-depth exploration of sexual intimacy is beyond the scope of this book, but I highly recommend the book *Come As You Are: The Surprising New Science That Will Transform Your Sex Life* by Emily Nagoski, sex educator and behavioral health expert, which will provide you with an incredible foundation for understanding sexual desire.

WHEN SHOULD I BE CONCERNED?

Most of us would be less interested in something we have enjoyed in the past if it was suddenly accompanied by pain, so addressing underlying causes of physical discomfort during sexual activity is incredibly important—and completely possible! If pain is at all a factor in your decreased desire for sex, read the "Vulvovaginal, Urinary, and Pelvic Floor Changes" section on page 105, and have a talk with your practitioner. Even if it's not a sign that you have a

Pleasure for One

The benefits of self-pleasure are infinite. Connecting with yourself through touch allows you to experiment and discover what feels best to your body—and you get to feel it! Physiologically, arousal and increased blood flow in tissue throughout the vulva and vagina is helpful for maintaining them long-term. Engaging pelvic floor muscles is a wonderful way to grow your awareness of how you can work with those muscles, plus it's a great way to both exercise and relax them.

Sexual pleasure can reduce stress—hormones released during sex reduce cortisol levels—and prompt an increase in serotonin, which can make us feel peaceful and relaxed. Another benefit of regular self-touch, albeit a less sexy one, is that you will notice if there are any changes to your body—a different texture in your breast or an unpleasant sensitivity in your vagina—earlier than if you were not exploring it regularly.

> "I'm actually hornier than I ever have been. Well, it started like in my thirties, I just started to get hornier, and then there have been times in my life where I've been more and other times where I'm not. But right now, I have to masturbate like every other day, or I'm just in a bad mood or I eat too much."—Maude

medical issue, it is very likely that your discomfort could be lessened if not resolved. Nagoski says that the only effective measure of your sex life is whether or not you enjoy the sex that you are having. Not how much or what kind, just enjoyment. Changes in your interest in or pleasure during sex, even with yourself, might cause you the kind of distress that comes with not feeling like yourself. Reach out to a counselor, therapist, or a close friend to discuss any persistent feelings of disconnection from yourself or your partner.

SKIN CHANGES

During perimenopause, you may experience a variety of changes to your skin including acne, hair developing in new areas (upper lip and chin), hair thinning where you still want hair, dryness, and wrinkles. Which of these skin changes you might experience depends on your age during perimenopause and your genetics, lifestyle, and environment.

CAUSES

Estrogen plays an essential role in keeping tissue throughout our body plump and malleable. In your skin, estrogen influences collagen production, skin thickness, and overall hydration. When estrogen declines, skin becomes drier, less elastic, and thinner, which can make it feel itchy and become less taut, showing signs of aging. Hormone fluctuations can also lead to the development of hormonal acne, which usually crops up around the mouth, chin, and jawline.

WHEN SHOULD I BE CONCERNED?

The skin is your largest organ and the only one that forms a physical barrier between you and the outside world. Keeping it healthy— protected and hydrated—is important to ensure that it can effectively heal any wounds, but also for your overall comfort. Any time you notice persistent discoloration or growths on your skin that change in color, size, or shape, you should consult a practitioner. Likewise, if you are experiencing persistent skin irritation like a painful rash or itching or acne that is impacting your quality of life, you may need expertise from a professional as you navigate an effective treatment option.

SLEEP DISTURBANCES

There are several ways sleep can be impacted during the menopause transition. Insomnia is clinically defined as a struggle to sleep that occurs multiple times each week for three months and negatively affects a person's experience of their daily activities. Sleep challenges can understandably lead to increased anxiety and, in some cases, depression.

CAUSES

During the menopause transition, there are many potential culprits for disrupted sleep: hot flashes and night sweats, hormonal fluctuations that cause changes in the sleep cycle or reduce the ability of the brain to calm down, age-related changes in metabolism (read: insulin resistance), a need to urinate, stress, medication, chronic pain, and sleep disorders like sleep apnea. Ideally, a practitioner can work with you to better understand the root issue of waking and staying awake during the night. Because there are so many possible causes—relationship stress, pets sleeping on your bed—a practitioner will probably ask you for some details about your sleep and other events and factors in your life that might be influencing your experience.

Some practitioners may ask you to keep a sleep journal for a week or two in which you track the time you went to bed, the time you woke up, and how long you were awake throughout the night. Treatment of sleep disruption will vary depending on the root cause(s) of the problem.

WHEN SHOULD I BE CONCERNED?

Sleep is becoming a more prominently discussed topic in mainstream media as research emerges about the importance of consistent, quality sleep for our overall health. You're probably familiar with the stock recommendations for seven to eight hours of uninterrupted sleep each night, but maybe you are less clear on what constitutes an "interruption." Most practitioners consider waking up in the middle of the night and falling back to sleep within fifteen minutes acceptable—not an interruption. If you are waking up, staying awake for an hour, and struggling to fall back to sleep, that would be classified as interrupted sleep. Sleep cycles can shift as we age, but if changes in your sleep begin to affect your ability to function throughout the day, consult your practitioner.

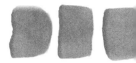

> "I had a baby a little over four years ago. Everything was fine, but I started having night sweats within a few weeks of getting back from the hospital, which is not uncommon as your hormones recalibrate. It was kind of gross, but I knew that was normal. Then it just continued. It continued for years, and it just gets very old to be sopping wet in the middle of the night—to have dirty, dirty bed and dirty, dirty body." —KRISTIN

VASOMOTOR SYMPTOMS: HOT FLASHES, NIGHT SWEATS

"Embarrassment all over your body because it's hot and prickly, but with even more sweating"—this is how one woman I interviewed described hot flashes. There is a range of sensations in hot flashes, including a slow or sudden heat wave that moves through your body, tingling or burning, and possibly a feeling of your heartbeat speeding up. The heat usually begins in the upper body, but you may feel it, and accompanying sweat, all over your body. Hot flashes can last anywhere from a few seconds to a few minutes. You could experience them intermittently over a few days or have multiple flashes within an hour. Everyone's hot flashes are different in how often they occur, their intensity, and how long they hang around.

When hot flashes happen at night and cause profuse sweating, they are called night sweats. It's the kind of sweating that drenches your sheets and nightclothes. Heavy sweating can lead to chills and shivering as your body works to normalize your temperature.

Hot flashes are like the prom queen of menopause; they get most of the attention, and there are some valid reasons for that. For starters, sweating through your sheets or having your temperature fluctuate wildly on the regular is disruptive. Sweat sounds innocuous enough, but it's not innocuous if it wakes you up and you can't get back to sleep, if it's accompanied by burning pain, or if it's trickling down your neck while your face is turning red and blotchy when you're in public.

Research data shows that 60 to 80 percent of people who go through menopause report having hot flashes during perimenopause or postmenopause. Hot flashes are typically the most intense and frequent during perimenopause and for the first one to two years after your last menstrual period. Information collected in the SWAN study showed that Black women report the highest frequency of hot flashes, followed by Hispanic, white, Chinese, and Japanese women. Approximately a third of all people who have hot flashes will have severe ones, and about a quarter of those people will have hot flashes over six or more years. People who start experiencing hot flashes while they're still menstruating (i.e., early in perimenopause) tend to have them for a more extended period.

CAUSES

Hot flashes and night sweats are called vasomotor symptoms (VMS) by medical professionals. *Vasomotor* refers to the nerves that manage dilation and constriction of blood vessels in response to signals from other sensors in the body to regulate your body's temperature. Your body likes to keep its temperature within a specific range, called the thermoneutral zone. Just like the thermostat in your house, when the hypothalamus notices that your body is outside of that zone, it initiates activity to get you to either sweat or shiver and bring that temperature back into the zone. Researchers believe that during perimenopause the temperature range the body deems acceptable

"I lost all kind of vasomotor stability, so any kind of stress, like in a meeting, or half a glass of wine, or anything would cause me to turn beet red. That is physically uncomfortable, and also emotionally uncomfortable if you're supposed to be the confident person in a room. So that was, in some ways, the most emotionally difficult part of the whole thing, because I just thought I was kind of crazy, it was often, and it went on for years." —DEANNE

narrows. As a result, the hypothalamus triggers corrective action—sweats or shivering—more often.

Without clearly understanding the mechanics of VMS, it has been challenging for researchers to identify specific risk factors. There is consistent data from studies in the U.K., Australia, and the U.S. showing that people with lower socioeconomic standing and educational attainment—both likely associated with higher stress levels—consistently have more VMS. Higher levels of body fat and abdominal fat in the earlier part of the transition to menopause and smoking or a history of smoking are also consistently associated with increased VMS.

> "My feeling with the night sweats and us all sweating is that we are detoxing for the next like forty to fifty years that we have—you know, potentially. It's like this huge cleansing, and so I love it. I love all the weird changes." —SHEILA

WHEN SHOULD I BE CONCERNED?

Both hot flashes and night sweats are most commonly associated with changes in hormone levels like those that happen during the menopause transition. They can also be caused by other conditions like insulin resistance, certain types of cancer, and thyroid or other autoimmune disorders. If you are experiencing hot flashes or night sweats at a point in your life when it is unlikely that you are in the menopause transition—that is, you are twenty-eight years old and have not had chemotherapy or an oophorectomy—you should talk to your practitioner. If hot flashes or night sweats are disrupting your daily routines in ways that impact your quality of life—not getting adequate sleep, too uncomfortable to exercise, increased anxiety—talk to your practitioner.

Heart palpitations, which can feel like your heart is racing or beating in some irregular way, are sometimes reported during hot flashes. If you experience heart palpitations, you absolutely want to check in with your practitioner, because while they could be innocuous, they can also be an indication of a more serious problem with your heart or a symptom of something like a thyroid condition.

There is research linking people who have frequent hot flashes and night sweats with an increased risk for cardiovascular disease, poor bone health, and dementia. While these studies show a correlation between VMS and an increased risk of these conditions, they do not indicate that hot flashes and night sweats cause these increased risks.

VULVOVAGINAL, URINARY, AND PELVIC FLOOR CHANGES

There is a name for the suite of symptoms that happen in these three areas: genitourinary syndrome of menopause (GSM). GSM expands on—and maybe slightly improves upon—the previous term, *atrophic vaginitis*, to include issues that arise because of changes to tissues of your urinary system and pelvic floor in addition to vaginal and vulvar areas.

Vulvovaginal changes could start with simply noticing that you can feel your vulva—a part of your body that usually waits patiently to be recruited into a feeling state. You might experience a niggling sense of pressure, or a bit of discomfort, dryness, or outright pain with any sort of vaginal penetration. Vulvar itching is also a common symptom. Note that vulvar itching can also be caused by an infection or skin condition, so if you ever experience chronic itching, it's time to visit your practitioner and discuss.

When it comes to the vagina, you may have heard the maxim "use it or lose it"—even from some medical professionals! First of all, ewww! What this creepy, vaguely threatening statement is trying to communicate is that, when the vagina or vulva are engaged in activity (which does not have to be sexual activity, by the way), circulation increases and helps tissues in those areas maintain

What Is Your Pelvic Floor?

Sometimes referred to as a "muscle hammock" running between your pubic and tail bones, the pelvic floor supports the bladder, uterus, and colon. When pelvic muscles are too tight, it creates one set of problems—constipation, inability to fully empty the bladder, pain during sex—and when they are weak, it leads to another set of problems—urinary leakage or prolapse, where the organs supported by these muscles drop down. The good news is that there a number of ways to care for your pelvic floor and keep it in good working order.

Kegel exercises, during which you squeeze your pelvic floor muscles, help you strengthen and maintain coordination of pelvic floor muscles. Learning how to do these exercises properly is important. For years, people told me that I could practice Kegels by stopping my pee midstream. Don't do that! Interrupting urination messes with your body; specifically, it confuses your nervous system. One way to learn how to engage and release your pelvic floor muscles is to insert your finger into your vagina (wash your hands first) and try to grip your finger and then release it. This exercise is helpful because we're not used to activating these muscles intentionally and having sensory feedback to see what it feels like can help you isolate the muscles. It's like the difference between imagining riding a bike and actually riding one. Once you've ridden a bike, you have what's called a sense memory and you don't have to think as hard about how to do it the next time you hop on a bicycle.

After you feel confident about how to do Kegel exercises, you can do them when you wake up and while you watch TV, do the dishes, brush your teeth, or any number of other daily activities. Relaxing these muscles is just as important as flexing them, so also consider practices like yoga, guided relaxation, and even breathing exercises.

elasticity. If you're experiencing vaginal or vulvar discomfort, it is not your fault. You haven't failed at sexual participation; your body is simply changing, which can be an unnerving experience. Though activity promotes elasticity, thinning tissue and a decrease in natural lubrication are not influenced by your level of sexual desire or activity. Even women who regularly engage in vaginal penetration can experience discomfort or dryness during peri- or postmenopause. These symptoms do tend to show up in later perimenopause or postmenopause.

If you are experiencing pain, whether it's during sex or not, a medical practitioner should be able to help you find relief within your boundaries. Lube during sexual activity and vaginal moisturizers

> "The most emotionally difficult aspect—I mean getting older is, you know, it's not super fun—but for a woman: losing the natural lubrication that we count on when we're turned on and that's just kind of there. But as you get older you dry out inside and that is, for a woman, I think not unlike a man being impotent." —DEANNE

are wonderful tools for anyone interested in maintaining vaginal moisture (for any reason). They are widely available, uncomplicated, and can be used with toys, vaginal dilators, and penises or fingers. Not everyone is interested in penetrative sexual activity, or sexual activity at all, which is completely okay.

Often people assume that if they are not sexually active changes to the vagina are inconsequential for them. However, if vaginal tissue is being affected, urinary system tissue will be too. Pain accompanying penetration may get your attention more readily than gradual changes in how often you pee or how effectively you can hold it, but all of these are indicators that hormonal changes are impacting tissue structure and flexibility. Urinary issues range from burning or tingling while peeing to a need to pee much more often, more urgency, or a bit of pee coming out when you laugh, cough, sneeze, or have a full bladder.

Unlike hot flashes and night sweats, GSM symptoms do not dissipate postmenopause; all but one (stress incontinence) get worse

STDs Aren't Ageist

Vaginal discharge, discomfort during sex, and pain with urination are all potential symptoms of sexually transmitted disease (STD)—or vaginal infections that are not STDs!—which is just one more reason to go see your practitioner if you experience any of them. Many of us tend to associate STDs with young folks as a result of our culture's presentation of sex as something that only young folks are interested in, but this is just not the case! If you are having unprotected sex, talking to your partner(s) about their sexual health—and keeping up on your own through regular testing— is a good idea regardless of your chronological age.

> "That's the other thing that started happening in perimenopause, I'd get up to go to the bathroom at three in the morning. I'm still doing that. I'm having more trouble sleeping, which could be pandemic, it could be changes in my own life, but I think it's compounded by my perimenopause."
>
> —AIMEE

over time. About 15 percent of people report GSM symptoms during their transition to menopause; 50 percent report some of these symptoms three years postmenopause.

CAUSES

Declining estrogen is the culprit of GSM, causing a thinning and drying of tissue in the labia, vagina, clitoris, bladder, and urethra. Estrogen keeps tissue plump and pliable; as it declines, the tissue in your vaginal lining and urinary system become less elastic, resulting in shrinkage and discomfort. This can also make you more vulnerable to bacterial infections because of the reduced distance bacteria have to travel to set up shop in your interior. Hormonal shifts also affect the pH of the vagina, which can make you more vulnerable to nonbeneficial bacterial overgrowth in the vagina and urinary tract, or yeast or other vaginal infections.

Bacterial Vaginosis

Many of us are familiar with the fact of the gut microbiome, the reality that both healthy and harmful bacteria populate our gut and intestinal tract. There is a decidedly less public conversation about the naturally occurring bacteria in our vaginas. It may surprise you that your vagina is a relatively acidic place, which makes sense considering that it is one of the few parts of our interior that we intentionally expose to things from the outside world. As hormone levels shift during the menopause transition, the vagina must recalibrate its bacterial population to maintain a protective stance toward incoming bacteria. In the same way that your gut bacteria and ecology aren't always victorious, sometimes the normal bacterial ecology of your vagina gets out of balance. A decline in vaginal estrogen leads to a decline in lactic acid lactobacilli that occupy the vagina. These changes create ideal conditions for bacterial vaginosis (BV) to proliferate. This type of infection can be experienced by women at any age, but as one of the downstream effects of menopause-related hormone shifts, a change in the pH of the vagina increases the possibility of an imbalance of bacteria.

Half of the people with BV do not have any symptoms. A pap smear would catch evidence of a bacterial shift, but for most of us, that test is—at best—an annual event. Suppose you notice vaginal discharge with a different texture or smell than you usually experience as part of your monthly cycle, or vaginal itching, burning or stinging during urination, or vaginal odor. In any of those cases, it's an excellent time to make an appointment with your practitioner.

Bacterial imbalances in the vagina can correct themselves over time, but BV is known for recurring within a few months, so many practitioners actively treat it. Conventional medicine generally treats BV with antibiotics; alternative practitioners might prescribe a vaginal herbal or boric acid suppository as a first step, followed by something to support and promote repopulation of healthy bacteria in hopes of preventing a recurrence. Most licensed alternative practitioners recognize the potential role of vaginal or oral antibiotics along with offering a strategy to restore vaginal ecology for the long haul. Depending on where you are in the menopause transition and the severity of your symptoms, your doctor may also recommend vaginal estrogen in addition to prescribing specific species of intravaginal bacteria. The vaginal estrogen helps to restore the normal lactic-acid-producing bacteria, restoring the vaginal pH and ecology.

WHEN SHOULD I BE CONCERNED?

Vaginal discomfort and an uptick in bathroom trips aren't indications of disaster, but these are signs of changes that are unlikely to resolve themselves without some kind of intervention. Bacterial infections in the vagina and the urinary tract tend to be persistent and can easily become a recurring problem, so consulting your practitioner is always a sound idea. Sex, with yourself or a partner, should never be painful. Although it may feel uncomfortable at first to discuss sex with your practitioner, that is the only way you can know with certainty whether your pain is an indicator of a more serious problem.

MISCELLANEOUS SYMPTOMS

There are numerous additional symptoms that people report having during the perimenopause time frame that could be associated with or caused by changes in hormone levels. Here are a few common ones.

ALLERGIES

Some people notice an uptick in allergies and asthma during their transition. Researchers have found that the hormonal fluctuation during the transition to menopause requires a considerable recalibration of the immune system; increased allergies could be connected to this added burden on the immune system. Though it might be challenging to pinpoint allergies as a menopause symptom, anytime you experience a shortness of breath or notice persistent wheezing or coughing while exhaling, reach out to a practitioner.

BLOATING

Many of you have probably experienced gastrointestinal shifts—bloating, constipation, diarrhea, or abdominal pain—throughout your menstrual cycles. As estrogen increases after ovulation, we retain water, which can cause bloating. Progesterone is also going up during this part of the cycle, and it has a calming (read: slowing down) effect on the digestive tract, which can cause constipation and/or bloating. Knowing that these hormones affect our digestion, we can understand what happens as they begin to fluctuate and decline. If you're experiencing chronic bloating, persistent diarrhea, severe abdominal pain, or blood in your stool, it's time to talk to a medical professional.

DENTAL ISSUES

Hormonal fluctuations have been connected to sensitivity in the teeth, swelling of the gums, dry mouth, and even a burning sensation in the tongue. There are receptors for estrogen and progesterone in oral tissue, so the decline of those hormones leads to thinning and drying. Deterioration of your bones, including the ones in your mouth, begins in your mid-thirties, and losing progesterone only speeds up that process. In your teeth, this can lead to increased sensitivity. Burning mouth syndrome, characterized by pain or tingling in the mouth that increases throughout the day, is experienced by approximately 2 percent of the population, but it has also been reported by people during the menopause transition. Dental changes can be indicators of other health issues, which is why seeing the dentist regularly is so important.

DRY EYE

Characterized by excessive tearing, a scratchy feeling, sensitivity to light, a burning sensation, or blurred vision, dry eye is most commonly experienced by women in midlife and is associated with changing hormone levels. Optometrists are likely to be more familiar with this issue, and treatment options, than a general practitioner or women's health specialist.

HOW DO YOU KNOW YOU'RE THERE?

You can confirm that you've arrived at menopause on your own if you track your cycle, because you will know when you've passed the one-year mark since you last had a period. Your doctor can also administer a test that measures your FSH levels, which will be elevated if you are no longer ovulating. However, FSH also fluctuates unpredictably in perimenopause, so it can be normal one day and elevated the next. There is a test that checks levels of anti-Müllerian hormone (AMH) because research has shown an association between specific AMH levels and the predicted time to menopause. Currently this test is used more frequently in evaluating infertility than in estimating one's arrival at menopause. If you are on hormonal contraception, all of this gets murkier; you will need to see a medical professional to help you determine if you've reached menopause and thus no longer need contraception.

The threshold to postmenopause can feel anticlimactic, in part because we generally do not have rituals to mark the occasion, but also because the symptoms experienced during the lead-up to menopause do not immediately disappear one year after your final menstrual period. To reframe the common (and cringey) medical terminology that calls menopause "ovarian failure," Gail Sheehy suggested in her book, *The Silent Passage: Menopause*, that we might instead think of it as "ovarian fulfillment" or the "gateway to a Second Adulthood."

"I talked to a medical doctor—allopathic, Western medicine doctor—and said I'm having this trouble and he said, 'Oh, you're too young for menopause, that's not menopause.' I was probably forty-seven or forty-eight or something. He said, 'That's nothing to do with menopause; that sounds like an anxiety disorder.' I was totally offended, but the interesting thing is that anxiety is not *not* a player. So, it's very, very confusing." —DEANNE

TESTING, TESTING, 1, 2, 3

Entry into perimenopause is trickier to pin down because it's a span of time defined by dramatic fluctuations in hormone levels within your cycle and in the timing and duration of your cycles overall. Many of the women I interviewed mentioned how nice it would be to know how long perimenopause would last or even how it would go for them. The not knowing is the characteristic of perimenopause that has the potential to make the transition frustrating, and possibly even destabilizing. It makes perfect sense that we want a test that could reliably answer the question we all have: What is my menopause transition going to be like? Unfortunately, that's not at all what is possible with the tests currently available in the market.

While verifying your hormone levels through testing sounds like a good idea at first blush, any measurement of hormone levels can capture only a snapshot of a moment in time, and it is impossible for you or a medical professional to know if that individual moment is a hormonal high point, low point, or somewhere in the middle.

Test results cannot capture the rolling reality of your hormone levels during perimenopause, and it is that variable production of hormones that leads to perimenopause symptoms. Ideally, practitioners diagnose and manage perimenopause experiences by completing a comprehensive medical evaluation that includes a review of your overall health and wellness, menstrual history, and any symptoms you report that you are experiencing.

Testing to assess the normal hormonal changes of perimenopause is done by measuring various hormone levels (estrogen, progesterone, testosterone, FSH, and anti-Müllerian hormone—a hormone produced by follicles in your ovaries) in samples of blood, saliva, or urine. These tests are costly and not always covered by insurance, and when used to manage menopause symptoms, they don't necessarily help medical professionals understand what's happening in your body substantially more than your own account of what you are experiencing. Symptoms are what helps your practitioner understand how your body is responding to this normal but erratic hormonal transition. If your body is struggling to adapt during this transition, it could be that hormones are going to be part of the process for getting you some relief, but testing the hormones in your body is not necessarily going to help the practitioner determine that.

Medical professionals are not in universal agreement about hormone testing as a clinical tool for managing menopause symptoms, and it is completely possible that you will get conflicting information if you consult more than one practitioner. If your practitioner recommends testing, before you commit it would be prudent for you to ask a few questions about how the results of the test would be utilized, how much the test(s) would cost, and how many times testing will need to be done.

If you're in your forties and you're having hot flashes and anxiety and your periods are irregular, a test that might be useful is a thyroid test, to make sure that your thyroid is not causing those symptoms. Unlike estrogen, FSH, and progesterone, your thyroid isn't peaking and plummeting throughout the day in erratic, perimenopause fashion.

If you are taking prescribed hormones to manage symptoms, testing can be helpful in assessing the effectiveness of the delivery mechanism (oral, gel, patch, and so on), but it is unusual for a practitioner to use results from a hormone test to determine *which* hormones should be prescribed or the dose of a prescribed hormone. However, some patients have complicated medical histories and issues of concern and thus need more investigative and management tools.

If you are on any form of hormonal birth control, whether via an intrauterine device (IUD) or pills, the estrogen and/or progesterone that your body would produce are being suppressed by the hormonal birth control; this renders any testing of sex hormones unhelpful. There are situations where a practitioner may want to gather more information because something about your specific situation is more complex, or to troubleshoot a hormone prescription that is not having the desired effect. The most important information to consider when exploring your options for confirming that you are in perimenopause or for managing your symptoms is what, if any, symptoms you're having, how often they occur, and with what intensity.

REALITIES OF POSTMENOPAUSE

None of us are defined by menstruation, but there is no doubt that our lives are influenced, if not altered, by its presence and absence alike. Our bodies are also affected by the end of our menstrual cycles and the hormones that defined them; normal, decreased levels of estrogen and progesterone postmenopause have a permanent impact on tissue and bone throughout the body.

Your new, lower levels of sex hormones, combined with the long-lasting effects of transition- and aging-related changes, impact your long-term risk for cardiovascular disease, osteoporosis, and dementia. Of course, there are other factors at play in determining your risk levels, such as genetics, health history, and environment.

Hot flashes and sleep disruptions can continue beyond menopause, and the likelihood that you will experience symptoms under the GSM umbrella increases as you age. However, uterine fibroids usually shrink after menopause, and a handful of perimenopause symptoms, like migraines and mood problems, tend to lessen and improve.

CARDIOVASCULAR HEALTH

Until age fifty, on average, females have a lower risk of heart attack and stroke than males. Females are in part shielded from plaque development, clot formation, increased harmful cholesterol, and decreased good cholesterol by their sex hormones. After menopause, decreased levels of those hormones means less protection for the cardiovascular system. There are numerous other risk factors for heart disease, including family history of cardiovascular disease, smoking, high blood pressure, high non-HDL cholesterol, insulin resistance, visceral fat, and type 2 diabetes.

Menopause and age-related changes in the body can elevate your risk for heart disease and a couple of conditions that contribute to coronary artery disease, which is the buildup of plaque in and hardening of the arteries that supply the heart. The clogging and stiffening of arteries can also negatively impact blood vessels that deliver blood and oxygen to tissues throughout your body, which can cause serious issues like strokes, damage to your kidneys, or pain in other parts of your body. Hypertension (high blood pressure) is a condition caused by microscopic damage to the walls of blood vessels that can lead to plaque buildup and stiffness, both of which force your heart to work harder to pump blood through smaller tubes. *Hyperlipidemia* (high cholesterol) is the term to describe having too many lipids (fats) in the blood. Both of these conditions elevate your risk of heart disease because they put strain on the heart muscles and diminish its ability to circulate your blood.

Stress is physiologically hard on your body, especially your heart, prompting it to pump harder and faster, which over time can lead to damage in the surrounding arteries. Although modern life is busy for most people, in the U.S. we are working more than we ever have and leading increasingly sedentary lives. Not only can the transition to menopause be a stressor but it can also often coincide with other life stressors like increased caretaking demands, work responsibilities, and divorce. Our bodies are naturally inclined to lose lean muscle mass and become insulin resistant during the years that, for many, are not flush with time for workouts and intricate self-care routines. Add all of these factors together, and you're looking at the potential for increased risk of heart disease.

Taking an inventory of your risk factors and mitigating the ones that are within your control—either via lifestyle adjustments or treatment options—can reduce your overall long-term risk. Most recommendations for heart health involve lifestyle adjustments, because research has shown lifestyle to be a better predictor of heart health than genetics (although if your father had a heart attack before age fifty, you are still at a higher risk for heart disease). Reducing or preferably stopping smoking is highly recommended, as is a "heart healthy" diet that is higher in fiber and lower in saturated fats and sodium, such as the Mediterranean diet. Getting adequate sleep and finding ways to reduce or manage your stress also tend to improve most aspects of physical health. Movement, even thirty minutes of it five days each week, will also go a long way to keeping your heart muscles healthy and your nervous system regulated. As Dr. Jen Gunter, author of *The Menopause Manifesto: Own Your Health with Facts and Feminism*, likes to say, "exercise is like free money, even a little is good."

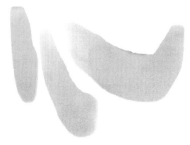

Women Don't Have Hollywood Heart Attacks

Inside and out, heart attacks look different in female bodies than male ones. We're used to seeing what's referred to as the "Hollywood heart attack," where a man gasps for air and grips his chest or paws at his left arm before stiffening and collapsing. Women are more likely to experience a persistent stomachache, nausea, fatigue, pain in the jaw, and breathlessness than chest pains. And if they do have chest pains, they are likely to be less crushing and more centrally located, with pain radiating down both of their arms.

Internally, heart disease in women tends to occur in the smaller blood vessels, not the major coronary arteries, which is the main area that doctors tend to examine. Angiograms, the test commonly used check for blockages in the coronary arteries, are not as effective in diagnosing women with heart attack symptoms because not all heart attacks are caused by blockages in those arteries, or any blockage at all. Women also have higher instances of heart attack caused by a spasm in an artery that creates a temporary blockage, or to have blockages in blood vessels that are too small to show up in angiography. The lack of visibility of these two potential causes has led to doctors' dismissing women with complaints of regular chest aches while exercising when it should be a signal that something more serious might be going on.

If you are having persistent chest pain, breathlessness, fatigue, or nausea and your doctor does not find evidence of blockages on an angiogram, keep pushing for further examination to determine the cause of your symptoms!

BONE HEALTH

Staring at a hanging model of a human skeleton and knowing the way our bodies are supported by our bones, it's easy to think of those bones as solid and unchanging. The truth is, our bones are dynamic, teeming with activity throughout our life span. Not only can they heal when broken, but they are also constantly being broken down and rebuilt in an effort to keep them healthy and strong. Scientists call this ongoing process bone remodeling. Your sex hormones play an important role in managing the pace of remodeling, specifically slowing bone resorption (the demolition phase of remodeling) and promoting bone formation (the building phase).

In your early to midthirties, you hit peak bone mass. Before that point, you undergo slightly more bone formation than demolition. In the years after peak bone mass, it is the exact opposite. When the breakdown outpaces the rebuilding, there is a net decrease in bone density that affects the strength and flexibility of your bones. Weight-bearing exercise does not improve bone strength or resistance to fracture during postmenopause the way it does prior to menopause; however, building up muscle at any time can help to support your bones, an added benefit to your overall health.

Osteoporosis means "porous bone," and it is the condition that leads to an increased risk of fracture; the highest risk areas are the hips and the spine. If you have a family history of osteoporosis and fragility fractures (especially in the hip) or have been a smoker or a heavy steroid user, your long-term risk of osteoporosis will be higher. You may also hear the term *osteopenia*, which basically means mild bone loss and refers to a natural, age-related decline in your bones. This term has been criticized by some medical experts who believe that it pathologizes aging and potentially encourages individuals to seek unnecessary treatment.

BRAIN HEALTH

If you experience brain fog and memory loss during perimenopause, there's a good chance that those symptoms will improve postmenopause. But the net downward shift in your sex hormones can have long-term impacts to your brain. We know that your ovaries and brain are connected health-wise because controls for body temperature, mood, energy, cognition, and sleep are all in the brain, and they are influenced directly or indirectly by the presence or absence of estrogen and progesterone. There is a growing body of evidence supporting the theory that estrogen is involved in processes that protect the brain from deterioration associated with Alzheimer's disease and other forms of dementia.

Having a family history of dementia or Alzheimer's disease will put you at higher risk, but other factors such as your environment, lifestyle, and medical history also have an enormous impact on the health of your brain. Caring for your brain looks a lot like generally following guidelines for healthy living: get adequate sleep, stop or don't start smoking, and eat a diet that fulfills your nutritional and energetic needs. Neurologists are digging deeper into the ways that the menopause transition impacts the brain. If you're interested in learning more about this, check the Resources section.

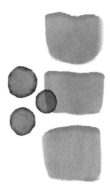

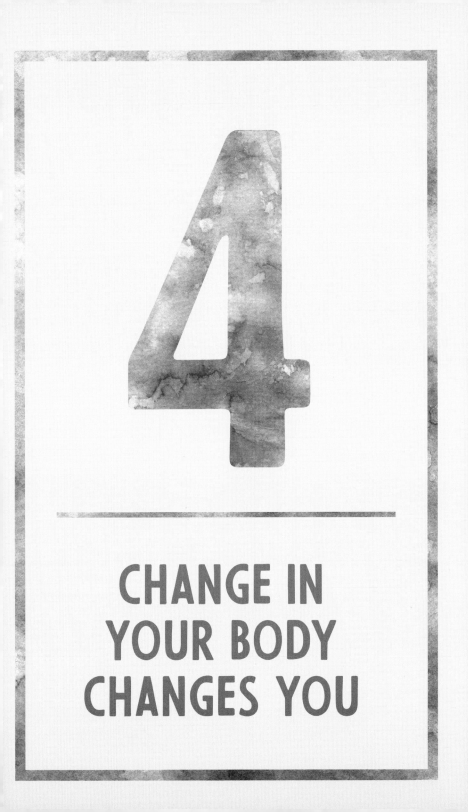

4

CHANGE IN YOUR BODY CHANGES YOU

Who is this woman going through the menopause transition? What are her dreams and aspirations? The answers to these questions are infinitely varied. Community. Vitality. Career. Family. Love. Movement. Mastery. You enter this experience at a unique point in your life, regardless of your age. You have plans and ideas for your future, you have people you love and feel loved by, and let's not forget, you also surely have responsibilities, whether to people, organizations, or causes (or all three). This life—your life—all happens in and through your body. Your body is a home of sorts, a deeply familiar place that is hard to isolate or separate from your experience of living in the world. Though your body does not define who you are, it would be hard to argue that the relationship between those two things is not integral to your lived experience. What is it like, then, when your body—the place that is integral to your life— begins to change, seemingly of its own accord?

"It would have been helpful to know that you get to explore your identity deeper as a menopausal woman the same way you did as a child becoming a woman. If that was part of what we're told that would be great, because it is. I notice my friends who are going through these changes, and they have to be more like we were when we were twenty in college together. They have to really think about who they are now, now that these things that have been working for them all their lives, things that you take for granted, don't work all of a sudden."

—MAUDE

WHO ARE YOU NOW?

Solastalgia is term for a kind of homesickness one feels when they are still at home. It's the distress one experiences when the place one calls home (their environment) has undergone significant change, has been degraded either by natural forces, colonialism, war, or climate change. Though the term was created to give a name to a kind of environmental despair, it is ultimately about feeling estranged in a deeply familiar place. When I first learned about solastalgia, menopause came to mind because it is a change (or series of changes) to the home you know and inhabit most intimately. Some of the changes in your body will influence how you move through the world and how it moves through you. Your confidence might rise up in new places or retreat in old haunts; your interests could stray into new territory.

"One thing that is challenging: typically when you don't feel like yourself or you feel sick or you have an ailment, it's temporary, and trying to wrap your head around whether changes are permanent or that you're sort of grieving; [you] didn't get a chance to say goodbye or really celebrate feeling yourself, whatever that is—that other person." —KRISTIN

We have this funny idea that we call the shots in our bodies, but the body is a force to be reckoned with. Anyone who has been mortified or inconvenienced by the side effects of something as commonplace as nerves (profuse sweating, explosive diarrhea, full-body trembling) can attest to that. Menopause is a reminder that we don't always have control, that we are aging and our that bodies will change no matter how we care for and tend to them. This can be a tough pill to swallow, because as we discussed earlier, we live in a culture (the social body) that believes aging is categorically a negative. Plus, change is disruptive, especially unprompted change within our bodies. For some, menopause is the first unequivocal reminder that time is happening not only out in the world or on their calendar, but inside their body too.

More than one person I interviewed mentioned that they didn't feel like themselves in some way: their fuse had shortened, they couldn't believe the words coming out of their mouths, or the things they used to do to keep up appearances just didn't feel like they mattered anymore. These shifts weren't necessarily upsetting, but I could hear a gentle crease of bewilderment on the brows of those recounting them. Though your ideas about who you are, what you do, and what you're capable of are not determined by your body, your body is essential to your experience of yourself. Changes in your body apply pressure to your beliefs about yourself and your habitual ways of being.

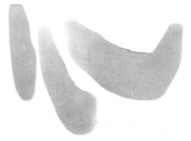

> "The biggest red flag for me has been periods of extreme lack of focus. Super frustrating when you're used to being able to focus on things and, you know, build your business and be a confident person." —JENNIFER

The intensity of an individual's emotional response to changes initiated by the menopause transition seems directly related to how much that change brushes up against the central pieces of their identity. You're likely to be challenged by changes to whatever aspects of yourself and your identity you've relied on the most: your mind, your looks, your energy, your calm demeanor. Destabilizing change has a way of illuminating what matters to us, whether that's a vision of the future we were counting on or a part of ourselves we've come to rely on more than we realized.

Many enter the transition to menopause in midlife, and in our culture, midlife is largely defined by what it's not: youth or old age. The dissociation of being neither here nor there can make it challenging to know what to wear, let alone where to set your expectations. Transition implies a certain in-betweenness, a liminal space where you're neither firmly in the place that you're leaving nor have you fully arrived in the place where you're headed. Liminal spaces, like the transitions through puberty and menopause, have the potential to make us feel liberated but also unmoored. It's easy to underestimate how disruptive that feeling of not knowing how to define yourself can be.

In midlife, for example, your role in your family may be shifting, with kids growing up and moving out (or at least becoming less dependent on you) or parents aging and becoming more reliant on your support. Job stability is a distant memory for most in our capitalist economy, and midlife is no exception, regardless of the type of work that you do. When clarities dissolve, you may have the urge to rush forward or yearn to go back to the way things were before you found yourself in flux. Midlife and other life transitions are not always tumultuous; it's just that the potential for disruption and uncertainty increases at this time. Author and organizational consultant William Bridges aptly describes change as a "low-pressure system" on the map of your life, capable of attracting storms and conflict, creating the conditions for old grievances to resurface and old scars to ache.

Visible changes in your body come with additional concerns. If you develop acne, move slower, turn red, sweat a lot, or develop a different body shape, it can change how you're perceived and treated by others. Self-love is not contingent on your body looking or being any particular way, but that's hard to hold on to in a society where judgment of bodies happens all the time and, whether it should or not, has consequences. I will never forget the day that my best friend's roommate told her how brave she was for enduring the arch of stubble above her eyes while she let her eyebrows grow back after years of plucking. It sounded ridiculous, but even at the tender age of twenty-five, I knew he had a point: people were going to notice and judge her for it. It's challenging to stay grounded in your sense of who you are on the days that you catch a glimpse of yourself in the mirror and struggle to recognize the person staring back at you, or when you experience an unfamiliar suite of sensations in the midst of your routine activities.

Your individual context, the details of your life, your attention, your threshold for discomfort—all of it will give shape to your menopause experience. It's not about being strong or weak so much as being who you are—with all your expectations, distractions, and constraints—and living the way you live, in your situation. Hot flashes, brain fog, and urinary incontinence do not have to be traumatic, and they absolutely can be. If you experience symptoms, you may be tempted to compare yourself to others as a means of gauging how well you are managing or determining whether or not the way that you are is okay.

> "A lot of my peers aren't going through this because their bodies aren't jumping into it quite yet, and so I'm struggling with being in a really different place than my friends." —KRISTIN

It's surprising how challenging it can be to make space for your own experience, especially when it looks different from what other people are going through. The urge to compare is understandable in a culture of norms and standards like ours, but doing so ends with you feeling either superior or inferior in relation to another woman, rather than you being in right relationship with yourself.

ALL FEELINGS ARE FAIR GAME

There isn't a wrong way to feel about menopause. Your mother-in-law says she doesn't even remember it, your aunt swears it was the worst decade of her life, and a famous person claims that it was an entry to a more powerful version of themselves. Menopause is like so many other life experiences—childhood, school, puberty, love, work, sex: a bunch of people go through it, and they have radically different feelings and stories about it. The diversity of experiences makes it hard to offer a definitive answer when someone asks: What will it be like? or How am I going to feel about it? There is no one answer to these questions, and more important, there isn't a *right* answer.

"I've heard a lot women [say], *I'm grieving the fact that I'm not being looked at or that I can no longer bear children or there's just a general grief in me that this is an ending at some point or getting closer to the end of life,* and to me it's not about any of those things. For me, the grieving has been like the grief that I haven't expressed in my lifetime that's just been holed up in places, that it's okay to let it go. There's a more complete understanding of life and its losses and its beauties that happens or has been happening for me." —AIMEE

Joy, rage, fear, relief, frustration, power, embarrassment, loneliness, pride, and sadness are just a few feelings menopause can evoke. Similar to menopause symptoms, you won't know which ones you get until they show up. "Positive" emotions like joy, empowerment, self-awareness, and strength are affirmed and encouraged in our culture. Unmitigated struggle like the kind that can accompany anxiety, grief, or depression is a wrinkle in the positivity narrative that our culture works tirelessly to flatten out with advice and platitudes about how to boss, breathe, or life-hack your way to "better." In our current paradigm, change is framed as an opportunity for transformation to which there is always an upside. This optimistic perspective can be inspiring, but it's also devious in the way it works to convince you that, if you're having a hard time, it's because you're doing something wrong. The thing is, change doesn't always feel like a win, and there is nothing wrong or weird or bad about that.

Change always involves loss or letting go; the changes that menopause brings into your life are no exception. Habits, power dynamics, routines, interests—all these things can shift as a result of or in tandem with your menopause transition. Some of the losses you experience will feel liberating, others may be devastating. Loss, and any grief that comes with it, is like a fly in the ointment of our solutions-oriented culture because it's not a problem that can be solved. Grief is one of many healthy and reasonable responses to loss of any kind, not just death and dying.

No matter what the changes are that arrive in your body and life, you will need to unwind the parts of yourself that were tethered to whatever it is that's ending before you can find a foothold for yourself in the new. This process will take time, and during that time you might feel impatient, excited, disoriented, free, or frightened. Perimenopause, like puberty, is a liminal time when you're in between two clearly defined developmental phases. The uncertainty of that amorphous middle ground can make you yearn for or grieve the loss of the familiar.

"There's an adventure-y quality to it, kind of like when you first get your boobs, you know [*laughs*]." —MAUDE

If you are having a great menopause experience, that's wonderful. There's nothing wrong with you (or better about you) if you're not struggling or uncomfortable. You might experience some resistance from your peers because *easy* is not a word we often hear associated with menopause. The other two bodies, cultural and political, have constructed confusing narratives of menopause over time, but *great* and *easy* do not feature prominently in any of them. Though I did not speak with many women who described the journey to menopause as enjoyable, the women who have gone through it had a clear message: there is indeed great living happening on the other side.

YOUR FEELINGS ABOUT YOUR FEELINGS

It's hard to tell which is the greater challenge, the feelings we have about something or the feelings, in the form of judgments and assessments of ourselves, we have about our feelings. Buddhists refer to this kind of self-judgment as the second arrow, the first arrow being the initial upset. I call it piling on. It is difficult to welcome, or even tolerate, experiences that are not what we hoped for or expected. Whether our initial feeling is one of unbridled enthusiasm or existential disappointment, we're likely to haul it into the interrogation room in our mind (the one with harsh fluorescent lighting) for evaluation and criticism. When our emotional response is different from what we expected, it can undermine our confidence that we know who we are. When our response is different from that of the people around us, we wonder whether the way that we are is okay.

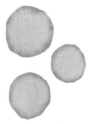

"A friend said, 'What you're going to find is that you want to be alone and you need to be alone, and it's okay to be alone.' I'm a very social person, so when that started happening, I was like, this is weird, am I a mean person?" —SHEILA

Second arrows are always whizzing around us, but they became even more noticeable to me during the COVID-19 pandemic. Once we were collectively swimming in unfamiliar waters, it became increasingly difficult to discern the difference between reasonable and unreasonable. What level of fear made sense given the situation? How sad was it appropriate to be; was it supposed to be relative to how much you'd lost? Were you using the pandemic as an excuse to not see your family? Were you an asshole if you enjoyed yourself or felt better than you had in months because you finally had enough time to sleep? What did it mean about you if you were wondering why you ever thought it was a good idea to live with your partner and have children? Those are all challenging thoughts to have. In fact, most of them are challenging enough that we would count ourselves fortunate if we could speak them aloud to even one person in our life. A lot of us didn't feel safe saying them to anyone because *what kind of person makes it all about themselves in the middle of a pandemic?!?*

Author Megan Devine gave words to something I'd experienced but never named in her book *It's OK That You're Not OK: Meeting Grief and Loss in a Culture That Doesn't Understand.* The Grief Olympics are that thing we do where we compare our pain or challenge or upset to the experiences of other people, often as part of a calculation to determine whether or not we are worthy of sympathy, treatment, or support. It can be overt, like when your cousin says, "You're only having hot flashes once a week—that's nothing! I'm having them all day and night." Or it can be more subtle like when your doctor tells you that periods are painful sometimes and asks you if you're sure that you're not just feeling a little overwhelmed and anxious.

The underlying presumption is that there is a ranking somewhere with all the variations of hardship and then what the person going through them deserves in response. It sounds crazy when you say it out loud, but it's a thing that we do in our culture, both to ourselves and each other. One of the reasons that the Grief Olympics is so tricky is because, when we reject the care and support that might make us feel better or heal faster, we often get rewarded for being tough, or at least we avoid being judged as weak. Those feel like wonderful accolades when we see them without their corresponding costs to us: the loss of time, the suffering or discomfort, the unresolved grief, and the sense of isolation that rides in lockstep with the pride of going it alone.

Secret judgments and concerns about the potentially horrible realities of who we are live rent free in our minds for decades, shame gathering in the nooks and crannies. There was a consistent pattern in the conversations I had with women about their menopause experiences in which, immediately after describing a difficulty (symptom or feeling), they would either tell me that they wished they were handling things better or that they hadn't figured out how to embrace what was happening to them. I could relate to their desires, and I also found it heartbreaking to listen to them layer a concern about not being adequately resilient on top of an already challenging situation. But that is what our culture teaches us to do. These conversations left me wondering about the standard against which we're evaluating ourselves: when it's okay to feel what.

"It's not like you can walk around in the grocery store and say, 'Hold on a minute, I'm having a hot flash, can you all come stand around me and hum? Let's just come together in the frozen aisle, please; I need your help, as an elder of the female community.' No, you have to figure out how to wipe your face because your mascara is draining down your eyes and you're wet and your body feels weird. It makes me sad, and I'm trying to get around this idea of *how can I harness this?*" —SARA

There's a lot of noise about menopause, and that can make it challenging when we have an experience that doesn't align with the dominant narrative or even just with what our friends are saying. Our emotions don't always make logical sense to us, and this sets us on our heels when other people ask us to rationalize things like why we are experiencing grief about the end of our fertility when we never wanted (and still don't want) to have children. Carving out space for your experience often involves breaking the habit of thinking, "I get to feel this way because someone (or everyone) says it's an okay way to feel." Menopause contains multitudes, and you're the one who gets to name what you experience. No one else has to agree with you or validate your feelings for them to be real.

OTHER PEOPLE'S FEELINGS ABOUT YOUR FEELINGS

Even if we do everything that we believe we are supposed to, things can still go "wrong." No one enjoys watching someone they care about—or even someone they don't—go through a challenging time, and there are two parts to that. First and foremost, we want the people we love to feel safe and good, and second, we want that feeling of comfort and security for ourselves. When people think that you're in a dark place, they're likely to keep trying to turn the lights on. We are often hustled (by others or ourselves) through discomfort, upset, and grief, and that hurrying tends to prioritize the feelings of the people around us.

Whether it's a coworker who tries to assure you that there is a reason (maybe a lesson) in the experience you're going through, the neighbor who gives you a pep talk about living in the moment, or the frozen smiles on the faces of your friends as they nervously avoid a touchy subject, the message is clear: everyone would appreciate it a lot if you could hurry up and get yourself back to okay. But not everything has a silver lining or is part of some master plan for your development.

As grief expert Megan Devine explains in her book *It's OK That You're Not OK*, "As a culture, we don't want to hear that there are things that can't be fixed." Sometimes stuff is just difficult and upsetting and not going to get resolved. Being there for people does not have to mean fixing whatever is at the root of their pain—which is great news considering how often we can't—but it does mean that everyone needs to be willing to wade into the awkward waters of not-okayness without an expectation that it will get better in the next fifteen minutes. In a world filled with *helpful* people, it's hard to remember that you are always allowed to have your experience at your own pace.

"I'm going to go into this as graciously as I can. I don't want to complain. I've been in meetings with people with handheld fans and I have heard the horrible stories about the dreaded sweats at night. I found myself looking at it the same way that I did with my cycle (this dreaded period), but every day is so beautiful and so not promised. I just don't even feel it right or righteous to look at a day with dread before that day has the opportunity to prove itself to you. Listening to the testimony of others had me in a space where it's like maybe I don't need to listen. Like am I hearing their wisdom or am I setting myself up, am I allowing their experiences to impose on my thinking?" —**ALATHEA**

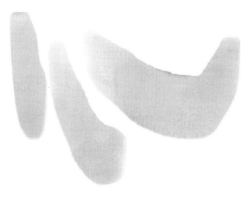

It's hard enough to remember that other people's reactions (positive or negative) to your feelings have little and often nothing to do with you, let alone to respond generously. In moments when I feel particularly prickly about someone's response to or interrogation of my experience, I try to employ writer Rebecca Solnit's practice of responding to closed questions or statements—the kind that aim to enforce or punish—with open ones: "Why does what I said surprise you?" or "I'm not sure that I understand what you mean; tell me more." Sometimes this is light work, other times it's a heavy lift, but most of the time it moves the conversation along and often back in the direction of the other person.

"I have a lot of respect for women who feel sadness around the fact that their period is ending and their fertility. I respect that that is some people's experience, and that is not mine at all. Hearing from women my age range who have internalized a lot of the messages about aging and worthlessness and you're sort of 'past your prime' or you missed the boat or the back nine—like all of those kinds of casual inferences that things that are coming aren't possibly going to be as good as what's passed. That hasn't aligned with my experience." —CHELSEA

WHAT COULD IT BE LIKE FOR YOU?

MAYBE YOU'RE FEELING CONFUSED

Confusion is a very real experience that we have, when we get turned around following a set of directions or when we lose the thread in a story for example, but it's also a tactic we employ when we want to avoid feeling something that we would rather not feel. I had an employee once who often said, "I'm confused," every time I changed one of our processes. The first few times it happened I fell into the trap of thinking that more or different information was the ticket to clearing up her confusion, so I added details, imagined scenarios, and reached for metaphors to help her see what I meant. My creative explanations never worked with my employee, because her confusion wasn't a matter of comprehension, it was a gentle act of resistance to something she didn't agree with (or just plain did not like) but also wasn't comfortable articulating her feelings about.

I remember how confusing the changes in my body during puberty felt to me and how little it helped to know that a shift in sex hormone levels was making breasts grow on my chest and hair spread across my pubic bone. The question that plagued me—Why is this happening?—was more existential than practical. The breasts and pubic hair were not really the problem; the problem was what I understood or believed that they represented and the fact that I did not feel ready to become a person with breasts and pubic hair.

Understanding that you can use confusion as a tactic won't change how you feel about whatever is the source of your confusion, but noticing when you're doing it does shift something internally. These days, when I hear myself saying, "I don't understand," I hear it as a statement directed inward, as if I'm telling myself that I'm experiencing something that I can't make sense of yet or that makes me uncomfortable. It doesn't always mean that I'll speak up and share the underlying feeling, but it does give me a way to stay with myself instead of checking out or overriding my experience.

If you're feeling a lot of resistance to or confusion about your menopause experience, it might be worth doing this two-part exercise.

1. Describe the place where you find yourself these days and what about that place feels so foreign to you. What's telling you that you don't belong? Is this a place you *ever* thought you would be? Are you dressed inappropriately? Do you not feel comfortable around the other people who are there with you?

2. Do you have a clear sense of where you thought you would be, the place where you would feel like you belong? Take a few moments to describe that place, and note how this place you imagined is different from where you are as well as any similarities between the two.

Sometimes this can help clarify the root of the disconnect. Understanding the root of your upset won't diminish physical symptoms, but it might offer some insight into where there's an opening to grieve something that didn't happen, or to connect with what's important to you moving forward.

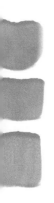

PART THREE

What Can You Do About It?

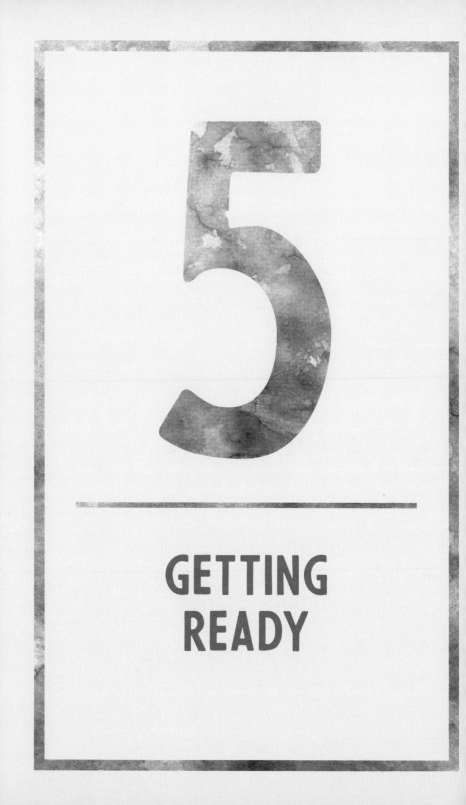

5

GETTING READY

Ready doesn't mean having certainty, being fully protected, or bypassing the process. In the context of menopause, I equate readiness with being aware of the forces at play—in your body and in the world—in a way that enables you to notice what's happening, call in the support that you need, and make decisions about how to proceed on your terms. Gathering information is the easy part; it's that next step of figuring out how to process what you've learned and apply it to your situation, your body, and your life that can feel intimidating. Understanding what could happen, how it might feel, and what you can do about it are important only in how they serve your capacity to identify aspects of your experience and access care and support that works for you. In other words, becoming knowledgeable about menopause is helpful, but getting to know yourself (your body and your feelings) is where it's at.

AWARENESS AND TRACKING

Fertility tracking always sounded to me like something for people trying to get pregnant. It is a great tool for that, but it can also yield a treasure trove of information about health concerns beyond fertility, such as thyroid disease, fibroids, and polycystic ovarian syndrome (PCOS). Tracking your menstrual cycle and symptoms is one of the easiest first steps you can take to prepare for your menopausal transition. Even if you capture a few months of data about your cycle, it can help you understand how the rise and fall of your sex hormones affects your body before those hormone levels begin to change. For example, you may notice that you have a lot of energy right before you ovulate (peak estrogen) or that you are always constipated right at the end of your cycle (lowest flow of both progesterone and estrogen), and these observations can offer insight into the way your body responds to the highs and lows of each hormone. The data you collect can also serve as a meaningful guidepost for measuring future changes.

Any time you're talking with your practitioner about symptoms, they are likely to ask you when the symptoms started and what kind of impact they are having on your life. As much as I don't want to add anything to anyone's to-do list, I also know that it's difficult to help and support someone until you gain some understanding of their situation. Having a record of changes in your body—mood, skin, cognitive function, sleep, digestion, body temperature, energy levels, and sex drive—is helpful both for you and your practitioners. Identifying what is happening, regularly and irregularly, in your body and defining what health or feeling good in your body means to you are things that only you can do. Trying to help you get relief from menopause symptoms without that information is like trying to get your smartphone to give you directions without identifying a starting point or a destination.

Cycle-Tracking Apps in The Post-Roe Era

As the landscape of reproductive health shifts in response to the U.S. Supreme Court's decision to overturn Roe v. Wade, you may have new concerns about where your personal reproductive health data is stored and shared. These concerns are valid, especially considering how challenging it is to be well-informed about which and how much data individual apps are collecting and with whom they're sharing it.

The convenience offered by cycle-tracking apps is something that you will have to weigh against the risks the data you're sharing could pose if it were accessible to organizations with objections to or questions about how you're living or what's happening in your body. Your level of risk is based on your geographical location and access to financial, logistical, and emotional support. Apps specific to reproductive health are not the only ones collecting data that could be weaponized against individuals seeking abortions. In fact, the data used thus far in legal cases against women accused of illegally terminating pregnancies has come from search and browser history and emails. Geographical location data could also be mined and used to harass or intimidate individuals.

If you decide that you're not comfortable using a cycle-tracking app, recording your cycles and symptoms in a note-taking app or document, like a spreadsheet, is effective and, if stored locally on your phone or computer, would require a warrant to be searched. Pen and paper also work for capturing details of your cycle and symptoms.

There are apps for everything, and perimenopause is no exception. If you've been using some kind of technology (app, spreadsheet, calendar) to track your cycles, you will naturally observe changes in the rhythm and volume of your flow. You can probably add additional columns, symbols, or comments to the tool you already use to capture new experiences. When I started having intense hot flashes what felt like all the time, I noted when they hit me on the Notes app on my phone. Once I realized that I was having hot flashes about every hour and they were bad enough at night that they were disrupting my sleep, I scheduled an appointment with my doctor.

Tech solutions don't work for everyone for a variety of reasons, so feel free to go analog with a little journal or notepad. If you have one of those 365 days of jokes or quotes or new words calendars on your desk, you could start a practice of noting any symptoms you experience on the back of a sheet when you tear it off and tucking the stack safely into a drawer. The goal here is to have as much information as possible at your fingertips rather than lodged vaguely in the recesses of your memory. Although the burden of diagnosing should not rest on you, the more information about your experience you can share with your practitioner(s), the better positioned they will be to help. There are over thirty-four symptoms that have been associated with perimenopause. You might experience none, a few, or just one of them, which is why it's helpful to pay attention to changes in your body, even the subtle shifts. Remember, practitioners know *the body*, but you are the expert on *your body*.

DEVELOPING A DECISION-MAKING RUBRIC

People tell us to make good choices all the time, but we aren't given much instruction on how to go about doing that. Research and data are positioned as the best tools for making good choices, but sometimes it's hard to find the data you need. Even when you do, you still have to figure out whether the information is from a reliable source, how it was interpreted, and if the amount collected was enough to make the totals statistically significant. Raise your hand if you remember anyone teaching you how to do even one of those things. What happens instead is that we go out into a world full of information from experts, our overbearing friends and relatives, and the SHOUTING on the internet—and try to make sense of what's real, what matters to us, and what the next most elegant step along our path might be.

If you feel like every practitioner, friend, and website is telling you something slightly different about the way you should manage your menopause experience, it's because they are. When you are getting diametrically opposed recommendations about symptom relief or the best way to protect your health long-term, you can feel less empowered to make your own choices than abandoned in a stew of information. There are times when, the more information you gather, the more insecure, overwhelmed, and judged you feel. Contradictions masquerading as options abound, and it seems like everyone is wagging a finger at you. Sifting through the advice and expertise, you can begin to believe that there is a right answer out there and that finding it is only a matter of making a thorough search.

> "I don't do well with hormones, so I've tried to find ways over the years to ride out the symptoms through herbs and acupuncture. To allow it to do its thing but have some relief from the intensity of the symptoms and its impact on my life." —AIMEE

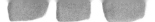

The last time I visited the integrative gynecologist, she sent me off with recommendations for a dozen supplements, and then after my blood work came in, a few more supplements were added to that list, for a total of sixteen. When I messaged her office with follow-up questions, like "Do I really need to take all of these?" the non-answer I got was, "You need to weigh the pros and cons for yourself if this is too much for you." Overwhelmed, I wondered if I'd been stereotyped somehow, pegged as a white woman in need of pills to soothe my perceived health anxieties, and I decided to take my blood work results to my general practitioner for a second opinion. I walked away from that consult with a recommendation to take just two of the sixteen supplements recommended by the gynecologist. Downgrading to just a couple pills a day was a relief, but it also made me wonder how I was supposed to know who to trust, given the spread between the two experts. I didn't want to be the idiot who took a bunch of pills I didn't need, but I also didn't want to be the idiot who didn't listen to their doctor and, as a result, wound up suffering from a preventable problem.

In the end, I went with a blended approach that was not grounded in any sound logic: I took only the supplements I had already purchased—which luckily included the two that both doctors recommended—and when those bottles were empty, I stopped. Without any evidence that I could observe in myself that the supplements were having the desired effect (or even an understanding of what that desired effect was), it was hard to feel motivated to invest more time or money in them. My experience with the gynecologist is not incredibly different from the experiences I've had in the twenty years since being diagnosed with a thyroid condition. Every doctor I've seen in the past two decades has a slightly different take on my lab results; at the two extremes, one questioned why I was on thyroid medication at all, and another urged me to take a barrage of supplements *in addition to* my prescription medication to support my compromised thyroid gland. I've been left to decide and advocate for myself based on my high school science education and internet search results.

Research—on herbs, supplements, hormones, pharmaceuticals, medical conditions, and tests—evolves and changes over time. It's incredibly difficult to make your decisions and anticipate their outcomes without too much attachment to their being The Answer. Health unfolds in ways we cannot predict over time, so we can only make "good" choices based on what we know and feel now. Knowing that you are entering a physiological transition where you may face questions you've never considered before—about medication, lifestyle modifications, and relationships—it might be helpful to have a method for navigating these decisions.

Economics professor Emily Oster has authored three books that center the decision-making experiences of pregnant women and parents of young children. The decision-making framework is inspired by the tools she offers to help people in understanding the underlying question they're trying to answer, how to find and evaluate the data they need to make that decision, and how to consider decisions in the full context of their lives. Although this kind of process-oriented approach to decision-making can make some people feel like they're turning their life into a series of calculations, having a bit of structure or a rubric can be helpful in the midst of uncertainty and overwhelm.

STEP 1: GET CLEAR ABOUT YOUR QUESTION

Start by clearly stating the question you're trying to answer. You might be trying to figure out whether a change in your body is being caused by the hormonal fluctuations of perimenopause or wanting to determine the safest and most effective course of treatment for relief from one or more specific symptoms. The goal here is to be as specific as you can be so that you won't be sitting down at your computer and typing *menopause* into the search bar. For example, your question might be something like: *This symptom is affecting my mood because it is preventing me from getting enough sleep, and I'm wondering if I should talk to a practitioner or just try taking something to help me sleep?*

Getting clear about the question is a tool you can use in the practitioner's office too. If a medication, supplement, procedure, or plan is suggested and you're not sure what it's for, you can ask the practitioner to help you understand or remind you of the issue they're trying to address with this recommendation. In chapter 7 there are examples of questions you can ask your practitioner to help you understand the path or process they're recommending you take. You can also work through some of the questions in the next step with them so that you walk away from your interaction with whatever information they can offer to help you make your decision.

STEP 2: GATHER INFORMATION

With your question in hand, it's research time. Using the example of a symptom that is causing undesirable effects, this phase will be more about identifying the specific effects your symptom is having on your life, learning about the symptom's relationship to menopause, and checking out common recommendations for addressing the symptom. You could do a mini-inventory for this symptom to assess how it is affecting your mood, work, family life, social life, and energy level. This is where any data you've tracked about your cycles or symptoms can be incredibly helpful! Keep things as simple as possible: nothing more than a three-point scale for these evaluations (i.e., 1 = not at all, 2 = a bit, 3 = a lot). You also want to make sure that you've noted any prior or current health conditions that may impact your risk profile such as a personal history of smoking, a family history of blood clots, or allergies to specific medications.

Once you're clear about the parameters of your current experience, you might talk to friends who've gone through menopause, check out information online, or even reach out to your doctor's office to give them the high-level view of your situation and ask what they recommend. It's also worth taking a pause to consider whether any of the treatments or approaches to getting relief resonate with you and seem attainable within your current situation, before you decide to adopt them. Even though symptoms might feel like they show up overnight, perimenopause is not an acute condition, and finding sufficient relief from the symptoms you experience can take time, as in weeks and months of time. Gathering information about how long it takes to see results with various treatment options is also important to help you set realistic expectations.

Before making a decision, examine all the information you've gathered, and reflect on your question. Sometimes you won't find as much data as you'd like or you will feel like none of your options are appealing, and that's rough. The only thing I can offer you in that moment is the assurance that it won't always be like that. Things are always changing—especially in your body—and the decision that feels and is the most right or wrong for you today may not be the best or worst one for you in a couple of months. There are some hard facts about menopause, namely that it is the end of your fertility, but the rest is well within the "let it unfold" category. Decisions about managing your health depend on many factors: how much you value the benefit you'll see long-term versus immediate gratification, how long you expect to live into the future, and your general tolerance for risk.

STEP 3: COMMIT TO A DECISION WITH CLEAR PARAMETERS

Pick a lane and commit. Be as specific and explicit as you can with yourself (and anyone else involved in the decision) about the desired outcome and how long you understand it will take you and your body to get there. If the decision you make requires significant effort on your part, it's helpful to set up checkpoints, which you can do with reminders on your calendar or using an accountability buddy. For example, I might decide I'm going to follow these four sleep hygiene practices for the next thirty days and note how rested I feel on a scale from one to three. If my rating doesn't stay at two or above during the fourth week, I'm going to talk to a practitioner about other options.

Patience and paying attention to any changes are crucial. It's understandable to want a fast-working fix that will restore things to order, and it's hard to predict what is going to work for your body and your set of symptoms in your circumstances. There are likely to be iterations and possibly even false starts in your treatment plan, and it will probably take time to see if it's working.

HOW LONG DO YOU WAIT?

When you're uncomfortable or distressed for any reason, a week is a long time, a month an eternity, and a year is inconceivable. It's cruel to chalk this thinking up to impatience because that doesn't take into account the white-hot panic you feel when you try to imagine how you're going to keep up with everything in your life now that you can't rely on your body or mind in the same way. Of course, it's good news that there are a bunch of treatment options that might offer you some relief, but you probably need more than a minute to wrap your mind around the reality that it might be a lengthy process—and maybe say a bunch of swear words or punch the couch—before you drop into that deep well of gratitude that everyone won't shut up about.

Before you start a course of treatment (prescription or not), check your expectations against these rules of thumb. If you've teamed up with a professional, ask them when you can expect to see results and what those results might be. Even if you're on your own, remember to make yourself a plan, preferably a simple one that includes how long you're going to do something or take something, a basic method of tracking whether you keep up with it, and what your metric for success is (meaning: what will "better" or "improvement" mean to you).

Rules of thumb for a few common menopause symptoms:

Hot flashes/night sweats: After four weeks of a given course of treatment without improvement, move on.

Chronic insomnia: After four weeks, move on.

Anxiety or depression: After four weeks, move on.

Cognitive shifts (i.e., memory and focus): Stick with a treatment for these for at least 2 or 3 months.

GIVE YOURSELF PERMISSION TO CHANGE YOUR MIND

Next, write yourself a permission slip that says, "I am allowed to change my mind, and I very well might do that." Knowing that you can change your mind eases the pressure around committing to a decision. If the decision you're making involves whether or not to take some kind of prescription medication, be sure to ask the prescribing practitioner about the process of going off the drug so you are clear about what kind of commitment you're making.

If and when you do find effective tools or treatments to provide relief from the symptoms you experience during perimenopause, keep in mind that employing those tools or treatments has potential to create friction in your day-to-day life. For example, developing a new bedtime routine to increase your sleep sounds like a lovely way to spend your time, and it also means that you will have to choose to take time away from something else. Your practitioner's recommendation for menopause hormone therapy to provide relief from hot flashes might give you that relief, but it also might make you worry that taking estrogen means you're giving in to the patriarchy. It's not easy to disentangle your physiological needs from your psychological ones. Taking time to understand why a specific approach does not work for you can help you identify one that's a better fit. Your odds of sticking with any treatment over time go up when all your needs are at least considered, if not met.

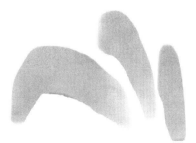

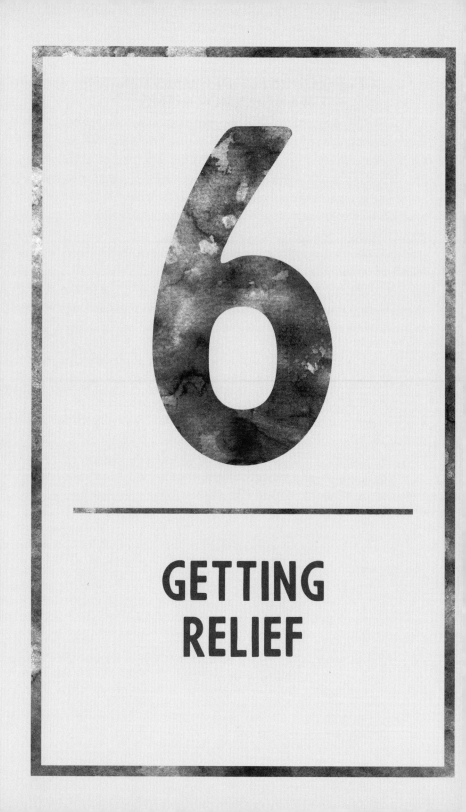

6

GETTING RELIEF

Although you can't sidestep menopause or control its timeline, that doesn't mean there's nothing you can do about it. There are a lot of tools, products, and low-tech solutions out there (like desk fans and lube) with the potential to make the symptoms you experience more manageable. This is great news! However, when you begin exploring, you may find the volume of options a bit overwhelming. Health is a complicated space in our culture, whether you're navigating it with a doctor in their office or on the internet from the comfort of your couch. Decisions about what to put in or take out of your body are influenced by many things beyond data from research studies. Fears about insidious marketing, hopefulness about safety and comfort, distrust of large institutions, and economic realities all factor into how you weigh your treatment options. Every medication you take, treatment you go through, or procedure you have poses some degree of risk alongside its potential benefits. The goal here is to familiarize you with current treatment options and offer some questions that can support you in determining which path will best serve you.

"I'm not saying [that menopause is] fun, but it is a powerful part of the walk and it's a part of the journey. I'm not looking for a bunch of quick fixes. I've heard of different things that people have tried and I'm not in such a big hurry to try a bunch of things, but at the same time I'm not in a place where any of my activities stopped as a result of my going through menopause."

—ALATHEA

THINGS YOU CAN TAKE

With any prescription for pharmaceuticals or recommendations for dietary supplements, keep in mind that literally nothing works for everyone. No one can tell you exactly what will work for your body and the set of symptoms you're experiencing without understanding your medical history and lived experiences. Yes, I'm talking about your friend or your aunt or your coworker who is urging you to take the supplement that is helping them with their night sweats or anxiety. Some of those personal recommendations might work, but they can also leave you exactly where you started, minus whatever you paid for the product. More important, be suspicious of anyone who has not reviewed your health history or current situation and tries to sell you a supplement that they swear is *helpful to all people* in the menopausal transition; the statistics are not in their favor.

PRESCRIPTION MENOPAUSE HORMONE THERAPY

If you have done even cursory research on menopause hormone therapy (MHT) and came out the other side of it feeling confused, you're not alone. MHT is the use of hormones to provide relief from symptoms caused by the transition to menopause. It is also a repository for immense cultural and political anxiety about women, aging, pharmaceuticals, and opportunistic capitalism. That's a lot of baggage to lay at the feet of one treatment! Do not misunderstand: There is not just one MHT; like "the pill" it has become an entire product category. Formulations and formats along with buzzwords to describe them have grown exponentially since estrogen was first isolated in a lab in the early twentieth century.

MHT is the umbrella term for treatments prescribed for relief of menopause symptoms, but practitioners may call it hormone therapy, hormones, estrogen, progesterone, or by any of the myriad branded product names. In fact, MHT was called *hormone replacement therapy* until recently when the term *replacement* was itself replaced because of its incorrect implication that decreasing hormone levels in women are evidence of disease or deficiency. As we discussed earlier, ideas about women becoming (even more) problematic and deficient—sexually, mentally, aesthetically—as they age have held sway for centuries. The North American Menopause Society's most recent update to their publication *Menopause Practice: A Clinician's Guide* demonstrates an interest in shifting our conceptualization of menopause: "Use of hormone therapy after menopause is considered therapeutic for menopause symptoms, not replacement for a deficiency state except in early or premature menopause."

Science, cultural beliefs, and capitalist interests have been pulling and pushing on hormone therapy since its creation. The point of contention has never been the effectiveness of MHT for offering relief to women experiencing specific symptoms (predominantly hot flashes and night sweats): that has been widely accepted for decades and is supported by volumes of data. MHT is a master class in the complexity of the interactions among the medical, cultural, and personal. Whenever there is a major change such as a medical breakthrough, a shift in gender roles and norms, or new social trends, everyone involved (practitioners, patients, and the public) is forced to reexamine their thinking about what menopause is, what it represents, and if and how it should be treated.

The first major shift in the use of hormones as a therapeutic came with the invention of synthetic estrogen in the late 1930s. This new source was easier to produce and calibrate, which resulted in more effective and accessible (to those who could afford it) products. It's worth noting that these early estrogen therapies came to market in the wake of miraculous drugs like penicillin that had dramatically shifted the public's expectations of medicine. The public began to expect that medical complaints could be resolved or cured with the prescription of a drug.

MHT (along with many other pharmaceuticals) was heavily marketed to practitioners in medical journals and via direct visits from pharma reps. It was also hyped to women (and husbands) in popular literature like magazines and advertisements. All these efforts by drug manufacturers created consumer demand, but there was still some debate among medical professionals, who did not agree about if and how menopause should be treated. Plenty of practitioners believed that menopause was a natural and normal progression in a woman's body and that reassurances of that fact were what she needed most.

> "One thing that's pretty mind-boggling to me is hormones. I mean, you go for help and it's kind of like nobody really knows, or they think they do, but every body reacts differently to it. This whole journey of balancing hormones, there really isn't clear information, it's mysterious. I don't know if that's a lack of research or if it truly is mysterious."
>
> —AIMEE

MHT has also had its share of medical missteps, like the increased rates of endometrial cancer that came with early estrogen-only formulations. Drug companies addressed this by creating a combined formula of estrogen and uterine-protecting progestogens. There have also been overreaches, such as the claim that all women should be taking MHT for long-term reduction in heart disease, which did not bear out in studies. Even with these serious issues, the fact remains that MHT has offered relief to millions of women from life-disrupting symptoms of menopause. Similar to every other drug (prescription or not), MHT carries risks, and the level of risk varies depending on an individual's health past, present, and future.

Anything you ingest carries risk. The amount of risk depends on your specific body, the amount you take, the route by which the medicine is delivered—oral versus through the skin versus through the vagina—and how long you take it. This is as true for bananas as it is for MHT; some bodies really don't work well with bananas, but for those that do, there are benefits to be had, including dietary fiber, carbohydrates, nutrients, and that taste! The difference is that the population of people eating bananas is a boon to the patriarchy, so the decision to eat or not eat bananas is not culturally contentious. Also, maybe people who believe you should only eat local food will shame you for eating bananas grown in another country and judge you for not being hip to environmental issues or workers' rights, but your decision to eat or not eat a banana is unlikely to challenge your identity the way MHT does for some women.

Current Thinking on MHT

MHT is widely accepted as an effective treatment for vasomotor symptoms (hot flashes, night sweats), genitourinary syndrome of menopause, and prevention of osteoporosis. Sleep disruption and mood swings can often be addressed effectively with MHT. There are a few scenarios where there is broad agreement in the medical community that the benefits of MHT outweigh the risks.

1. If you:
   become menopausal before age forty (aka premature menopause)

   become menopausal between forty and forty-five (aka early menopause)

   go through surgical menopause (aka removal of both ovaries)

   In these scenarios, if MHT is taken until at least age fifty-one (and possibly until death for those in surgical menopause), you will benefit from the preventative effect that MHT has on long-term health issues like heart disease, osteoporosis, and dementia.

2. If you do not have a history of breast cancer and are starting MHT before the age of sixty, less than ten years past menopause, and/or are experiencing vasomotor or other menopause-related symptoms that are negatively affecting your quality of life

But what about breast cancer, strokes, and heart attacks? If you've been warned about these specific dangers related to MHT, it's probably the downstream effect of a large-scale study conducted in the early 2000s called the Women's Health Initiative (WHI). The study was designed to test whether MHT played a role in the long-term reduction of heart disease that clinicians had observed in their patients. Researchers wanted to test both estrogen-only and estrogen-progestin (synthetic progestogen) combination therapies, so there were two tracks of the study running simultaneously. The short version of this story is that each track was stopped earlier than scheduled, and the communications about the reasons why were bungled. Headlines that ran in national media read like warning labels: "Hormone therapy increases risk of heart attack, stroke, and cancer."

On closer inspection of both the study and the resulting data, researchers segmented data by age range, and when they looked at the numbers for participants under age sixty, MHT did protect against heart disease and was also associated with lower risk of dying from any cause. Similarly, the data on breast cancer was more nuanced than initially understood. Women on an estrogen-progestin combination had a very, very slight risk of breast cancer after three to four years of use, while those on estrogen alone had less than a slight risk, if any at all. In addition, three other observational studies out of France demonstrated that women taking estrogen and progesterone (the bio-identical form often called "natural progesterone") had no increased risk of breast cancer.

As we have seen with communications about public health measures throughout the COVID-19 pandemic, data is complex, and even once we do understand the numbers, there are other forces (cultural, political, and personal) that influence decision-making.

Once a headline is out there with partial or incorrect conclusions, it takes a tremendous amount of work to undo the impacts of that message.

In conclusion, MHT does carry a slight to small risk. As I mentioned earlier, the variability of that risk is a result of our genetic snowflake-ness and lived experiences. The key risks currently associated with MHT are as follows:

1. If you have a history of estrogen-positive cancer, taking estrogen poses some risk of fueling that cancer. Note that, if you have a history of breast cancer and are experiencing GSM symptoms, you could consider asking your practitioner about formulations and forms of MHT (like vaginal rings or suppositories) that could be effective at managing your symptoms without increasing your risk of breast cancer.

2. A family history of cardiovascular disease or a personal history of clotting or deep vein thrombosis or heart attack puts you in a higher risk category for taking estrogen, especially oral estrogen. It is generally considered safe to take transdermal estrogens (creams, gels, and patches) and completely safe to take the low-dose vaginal estrogen for GSM.

3. If you are over age sixty or ten years past menopause, experts agree that the risks of starting MHT outweigh the benefits.

The Paradox of Choice

Prescribing hormones is a combination of science and art where practitioners are aiming to provide just the right amount of what your body needs when your body needs it while your body is undergoing dynamic fluctuations in hormone levels. The volume of MHT products on the market is, at least in part, a response to the need for very specific solutions for individual bodies, as well as consumer preferences. There are three primary categories of MHT formulations: estrogen-only therapy, estrogen-progestogen therapy, and estrogen therapy plus estrogen agonists/antagonists (also known as TSEC, tissue selective estrogen complex). Within these categories there are myriad variations, not just in the delivery methods (cream, pill, patch, etc.), but also in the individual ingredients (bioidentical, nonbioidentical, synthetic, natural), the schedule (continuous, cyclic or sequential, cyclic combined), the dose, the combination of hormones, where it goes in your body (local, systemic), and the way it is produced (compounded by a pharmacy or manufactured by a pharmaceutical company).

While the variety is overwhelming, your practitioner should walk through the most suitable options based on your needs and preferences. Factors to consider in selecting a specific product include the symptom(s) you're trying to address; known health risks including allergies, lifestyle, and product parameters you're committed to such as no additives; specific production or inspection protocols; and cost. It's also important to think pragmatically about your habits and routines. Some people will struggle to remember to put their patch on two times a week, take a pill every single day (there are different MHT schedules, just like there are for hormonal birth control packs), or apply cream every other evening. These are important realities to consider when your practitioner is writing you a prescription. I've heard more than one dermatologist respond to requests for recommendations on the best sunscreen by saying, "The one that you'll consistently wear." One thing we know for certain is that MHT will not help you at all if you're not using it.

If you are exploring MHT you will find that not everyone will agree with your choice to consider it, the kind you might take, the dosage your practitioner prescribes, and whether you get a formulation from a major drug company or have one made at a compounding pharmacy. We are living in the shadow of a complicated history that continues to inform our opinions of and experiences with the entire medical enterprise, including practitioners, researchers, wellness influencers, and pharmaceutical companies. It is always within your right as the patient to ask your practitioner to walk you through the decision-making behind their recommendation. If all you get in response is a stack of MHT brochures from pharmaceutical companies with an offer to answer any questions you may have later, it might be time to find a different practitioner.

Questions about MHT are warranted, not because this class of medication is inherently dangerous, but because medical and cultural attitudes surrounding MHT have fluctuated dramatically within our lifetime. Our understanding of the mechanics of MHT and of the symptoms associated with the menopause transition will deepen over time through continued research, cultural shifts, and medical practices.

Testosterone and Menopause

Androgens are "male" sex hormones that are also present in cisgender women's bodies, although in much smaller amounts (about one tenth as much). Testosterone is the main androgen, and it's commonly linked to sexual desire and capacity for arousal and/or orgasm, but it also may help maintain muscle and bone strength. Androgen levels decline as women age; this is unrelated to the menopause transition, but levels are clearly lower after menopause than before. Women who go through early menopause or surgical menopause as a result of a bilateral oophorectomy (removal of both ovaries) will also have lower androgen levels because testosterone is produced by the ovaries and adrenal glands.

Sexual desire is complex and layered, which makes determining the cause of its decline challenging. In addition, the majority of the research on the use of testosterone to address a decline in sexual desire is in postmenopausal women and women who are taking estrogen plus testosterone. Your practitioner should consider chronic depression, relationship issues, medications, stressors, physical factors (including other health conditions like fatigue, chronic pain, and pain with vulvar/

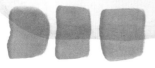

vaginal touch), and environmental factors alongside potentially testing testosterone levels (which is challenging because it's difficult for lab tests to detect very small amounts of the hormone). Testosterone medication could be part of a treatment plan for a decline in sexual desire and capacity for arousal and orgasm; however, prescription testosterone products are not currently available for women in the U.S. through conventional pharmacies, with the exception of one combination estrogen-testosterone pill manufactured by Big Pharma. Compounded testosterone, with and without the other hormones, is an option with a compounding pharmacy and a well-thought-out prescription.

MHT Keywords

There is a lot of terminology related to MHT. Here are a few of the terms you will hear most often.

Bioidentical: This refers to laboratory-produced hormones that are made from a compound extracted from Mexican wild yam or soybeans and that are virtually identical in chemical structure to their counterparts in the human body. Bioidentical does not indicate anything about the quality of the source materials, and the term is not synonymous with compounded.

Compounded: Compounded MHT is necessary for individuals who have allergies to additives in the MHT manufactured by Big Pharma and for those instances where the specific dosages, hormone combination, or form (i.e., sublingual lozenges, creams, capsules, or suppositories) that is prescribed is not commercially available. These offerings also appeal to people who want to avoid dyes, preservatives, and chemical stabilizers typically found in conventional products. Compounded MHT is produced and regulated differently than FDA-approved MHT.

Natural: This term is not regulated; it is essentially a marketing term. *Natural* does not mean more or less safe, it doesn't confirm that a product is regulated, and it is not synonymous with *bioidentical*.

Progestogens: This is the umbrella term for a specific class of hormones that includes progesterone and progestins. Progesterone is bioidentical, progestins are synthetic, and both are in the family of progestogens.

SERM: Short for *selective estrogen receptor module*. SERMs can be combined with estrogen to make drugs called tissue selective estrogen complexes (TSECs). TSECs are a type of MHT that offers the benefits of estrogen in certain tissues while protecting other tissues in the body from estrogen. These can be beneficial for people who are sensitive to progestogens but are seeking relief from menopause symptoms and still need to protect their uterus.

Synthetic: These compounds have chemical structures that are similar to human hormones, so they are able to bind to specific desired hormone receptors in the body. Synthetic compounds can be extracted from plants or from nonnatural sources and are made in manufacturing laboratories.

Systemic: This refers to a dose or delivery mechanism of MHT such that the hormones access tissue throughout the body rather than being restricted to a localized area. Oral systemic MHTs first pass through the liver, which presents risks for people with nonalcoholic fatty liver disease (because it can raise triglycerides or insulin resistance), hyperlipidemia, or a history of blood clots or deep vein thrombosis. Transdermal estrogens, such as patches and creams, and vaginal systemic estrogens do not increase the risk of these problems.

OTHER PRESCRIPTION OPTIONS

Low-Dose Hormonal Birth Control

Approaching the end of fertility and being infertile are different in one very important way: during the first one you can still absolutely get

pregnant. During the menopause transition, if you are not trying to conceive, you will need to continue to use some form of contraception during penis-in-vagina (PIV) penetrative sex. Oral and implanted contraceptives and IUDs do not offer protection from STDs, so that is a risk that you will need to continue to consider in your sexual interactions.

Low-dose hormonal contraceptives have higher amounts of hormones and different varieties of estrogen and progestogens than the highest dose of menopause hormone therapy. These (low-dose) formulations came about over time through efforts to provide effectively suppressed ovulation while minimizing the risk of blood clots and nuisance effects like breast tenderness, mood swings, and migraines. It can be a little bit easier to control bleeding during perimenopause with low-dose hormonal contraceptives than with MHT specifically because the dosage is higher.

Antidepressants

These medications make serotonin (SSRI) and serotonin and norepinephrine (SNRI) more available in the brain by blocking the nerve cells that normally reabsorb them. Both can be helpful during the menopause transition for managing depression or ongoing anxiety. For anyone concerned about hormones or with a breast cancer diagnosis, these drugs offer a nonhormonal option for addressing vasomotor symptoms. One possible side effect of these medications is diminished desire for sex and capacity for orgasm; this is an example of the many reasons why it's important to consider all of your symptoms when exploring treatment options.

Anti-Seizure Medications

People experiencing vasomotor symptoms may get some relief from them with an anti-seizure medication. This type of medication has been effective in helping people who are experiencing night sweats that are disrupting their sleep. Gabapentin is the most well-known medication in this category. At higher doses they can cause side effects such as drowsiness, dizziness, and headache, but relief from vasomotor symptoms can usually be achieved with a low dose.

NONPRESCRIPTION TREATMENT OPTIONS

It is not an overstatement to say that nonprescription options (dietary supplements and over-the-counter drugs) are, like prescription options, a locus of conflict in our beliefs about health, safety, regulation, and capitalism. Depending on your practitioner, anything you'd like to take to manage some or all of your menopause symptoms —prescription or not—could be either encouraged or discredited.

Many people have told their stories of frustration with practitioners who seem quick to offer them prescription medication without much accompanying explanation about the root cause of a particular symptom or ailment. Antidepressants, for example, are commonly offered to women when they report experiencing pain or difficulty sleeping. I have found the zone of nonprescription options to be no less confusing than that of prescription drugs. There are tools for relief from menopause symptoms in both categories, and yet you are likely to encounter conflicting reports about all of them, even if only anecdotal ones. Before taking anything, it's wise to seek out information about any contraindications (that's medical speak for health conditions or other substances that may make the drug or supplement you're taking do something you don't want it to do), especially if you are aware of any other personal health considerations or are taking other medications.

Most conventional practitioners are not adequately trained or informed on dietary supplements (vitamins, minerals, amino acids, and herbs), especially for perimenopause and menopause. Ideally, you would consult a licensed naturopathic physician or integrative conventional practitioner who is trained and experienced in the specialty of perimenopause and menopause and understands the full spectrum of therapeutics: lifestyle, dietary supplements, MHT (conventional and compounded), and other pharmaceuticals. Virtual healthcare (aka telemedicine) offers hope that this kind of practitioner will be more broadly accessible—and covered by health insurance providers—in the not-so-distant future.

Dietary Supplements

All nonprescription products formulated from plants (also called botanicals), minerals, amino acids, or vitamins legally fall under the umbrella of dietary supplements. This category of product is not regulated by the FDA in the same way as pharmaceutical products, although they are regulated by the FDA under the Dietary Supplement Health and Education Act of 1994 (which defined the term "dietary supplement" and allowed the FDA to define and enforce Good Manufacturing Practices for products with that label). Dietary supplements are distinct from drugs and as such are not allowed to make specific health-benefit claims. However, they can be labeled with buzzwords like *superfood* and *natural* that consumers have positive associations with but that do not have established definitions. There is a history of contention between the FDA and manufacturers of dietary supplements, with court battles over language used on product labels and deep-seated frustration that stems from a piece of legislation passed by Congress in 1994 that took away much of the FDA's regulatory authority over this category of products.

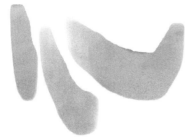

WHAT CAN YOU DO ABOUT IT?

Dietary Supplement Primer

Vitamins: These are organic substances that occur naturally in some foods and also are produced within our bodies. We need vitamins to help regulate metabolic processes—breaking down foods we consume into usable components. Vitamins are taken not only for the purpose of reaching the recommended daily minimum; there is a history of using individual vitamins and minerals in therapeutic doses for treating specific conditions and reducing the risk of select diseases, like the use of folic acid during pregnancy to prevent serious birth defects like spina bifida. A number of vitamins have health risks associated with oversupplementation, so be sure that you are taking the amount recommended by your doctor or cited in the national Recommended Dietary Allowance guidelines.

Multivitamins: These are combinations of vitamins and minerals designed to suit a variety of nutrient needs. Ideally you would meet your nutrient needs through your diet, but there are situations in which your diet may be restricted or somehow insufficient, and in those cases a multivitamin can be a helpful support. If you're taking a multivitamin and any other dietary supplements, you might want to review all the ingredients to ensure you're not taking more than you need of any specific vitamin or mineral.

Botanicals: Plants have been used as medicine for centuries. The primary considerations with botanicals have to do with purity and strength of ingredients, because plants can absorb toxins through the soil where they are grown, and individual botanical supplements also can vary wildly in their potency of the active ingredients.

Minerals: Like vitamins, these are naturally occurring substances that you would ideally get in adequate amounts from your diet, because the foods that contain important minerals are likely to provide more than one nutrient. Examples of common mineral supplements are calcium, iron, magnesium, and zinc. Minerals can be used in therapeutic doses to treat specific conditions and reduce the risk of select diseases.

Specialty supplement formulations: This category is enormous because it includes all the specialized formulations intending to address issues with sleep, metabolism, sexual desire, all of menopause, mood, energy, vasomotor symptoms, and your vagina. Beyond addressing perimenopause and menopause symptoms, there are also products designed to reduce the risk of conditions like osteoporosis, cardiovascular disease, and diabetes.

Dietary supplement manufacturers are no longer subject to the requirements and restrictions that apply to food, prescription or over-the-counter drugs, and medical devices. In 2007 the FDA created a set of safety guidelines to help manufacturers manage the quality, purity, and strength of their products, but unlike drug manufacturers, these companies are not required to provide evidence that dietary supplements are safe or effective for their recommended use. The manufacturers of dietary supplements are responsible for making sure that their product labels provide accurate and adequate information for consumers to make informed decisions, and that the dosage guidance is appropriate.

Although the FDA can step in if there are reports of safety issues after the product is on the market or if they find problematic information in published product information, the FDA does not even verify that supplements contain what they say they do. One way to identify manufacturers who are engaged in some level of quality control testing for their products is to search for labels with a USP, NSF, Consumer Lab, or UL verified logo.

There are examples of supplements with a demonstrated track record for positive health outcomes, like the use of folic acid throughout pregnancy to reduce the likelihood of serious birth defects. However, there is research showing that people who take dietary supplements tend to be healthier overall—better diet, more exercise, less smoking—and have higher incomes and higher levels of education; all these factors make it tough to attribute positive outcomes to individual supplements. Although the evidence of the effectiveness of dietary supplements varies considerably, their popularity persists because sometimes they work. Dietary supplements are another hotly debated topic among health professionals, with some practitioners arguing that the evidence showing that supplements are unlikely to do harm is not a reason to take them, and other practitioners saying that the low risk and low cost of most supplements plus the potential for even modest benefits make them worth taking. We, the consumers, are left to consider the available data and the recommendations we receive from trusted sources to make a choice that suits the health outcomes we're seeking as well as our full health history, risk tolerance, and budget.

If you're interested in working with nonpharmaceutical options for relief from menopause symptoms, you have ample options. The following chart is a list of the dietary supplements that have the most research supporting their effects on specific symptoms. Nearly every summary of these supplements will come with a note of caution reminding you that these products are not regulated in the same way as pharmaceuticals and that they have the potential for negative interactions with other medications. You should consult your practitioner (ideally one who is trained and knowledgeable in these botanicals and nutrients) before you take any of these. In addition to the supplements in the chart, calcium, magnesium, vitamin D, B vitamins, and fish oil offer benefits to areas of your body that are impacted by the menopause transition (and aging in general), such as your bones, brain, and cardiovascular system.

DIETARY SUPPLEMENT	USE WHEN YOU'RE EXPERIENCING . . .	NOTES
Ashwagandha	Chronic insomnia	Particularly good for those experiencing elevated stress and/or anxiety, whether it's related to the cause of the insomnia or the result of it. This is not going to help you with sleep immediately: it takes several weeks to have a regulating effect on the sleep cycle.
Black cohosh	Hot flashes/night sweats Mood changes Breast tenderness	Considered safe for breast cancer patients/survivors.
Evening primrose oil	Night sweats	In research, it has been helpful for diminishing night sweats but not effective for daytime hot flashes.
Ginger	Dysmenorrhea (uterine cramping, painful periods) Heavy menstrual bleeding	First, rule out other potential causes of heavy menstrual bleeding like thyroid disorder, uterine polyp, uterine fibroids, adenomyosis, uterine pre-cancer or cancer, and von Willebrand disease. Menstrual cramps can be just physiologic (called primary dysmenorrhea), which is what ginger is known to help; they can also be due to endometriosis or adenomyosis—ginger may or may not help cramps in those circumstances.
Kava	Anxiety disorder Hot flashes/night sweats	

DIETARY SUPPLEMENT	USE WHEN YOU'RE EXPERIENCING . . .	NOTES
L-theanine	Difficulty sleeping General anxiety	
Maca	Decreased sexual desire Fatigue Hot flashes/night sweats	
Melatonin	Difficulty sleeping	
Red clover	Hot flashes/night sweats Depression	
Rhodiola	Anxiety Depression Fatigue Other mood changes	If these symptoms are experienced in combination with hot flashes, a recent research study shows that combining black cohosh with rhodiola has improved outcomes.
St. John's wort	Depression Hot flashes/night sweats	
Valerian root	Anxiety Difficulty sleeping Hot flashes	

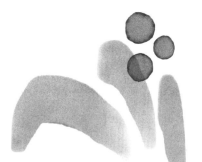

THINGS YOU CAN DO

The common thread running through everything in this category is time. All the following recommendations require it, and unfortunately not everyone going through menopause has the same quantity of it to spare. A friend once commented that one nice thing about getting older is that the answer to the question of "What's important here?" is clearer. While I agree completely, knowing what's important doesn't alter the constraints you might be living within—economic, logistical, or emotional—that can limit your ability to tend to what's important. All the activities and inactivities included here have varying levels of cultural acceptance and social currency depending on your geography, class, and cliques. None are better than the others, but some are probably better suited to address your needs.

If you have a tendency to turn leisure into labor, be mindful of that as you explore ways of taking care of yourself. It's easy to allow a low-key activity you started for relaxation (gardening, dance, crafts, cooking) to become another arena for competition and comparison—or maybe even a side hustle? Sometimes that is a completely natural progression, but for some people it's more of a habit. Investing time in yourself, especially when it's not pegged to increasing your productivity (yes, I'm even talking about self-improvement!), is hard for many of us to justify because it goes against the thrum of *always be optimizing*. Maybe pretend that you're asking yourself "for a friend" what might feel good right now, and then try your darnedest not to judge the answer. In addition, you can't (and shouldn't) try to change everything all at once. Baby steps are a great place to start, and honestly, with a healthy dose of patience, they can even get you all the way to your destination.

LIFESTYLE CHANGES

These are all the things that are easy to say and hard to do. The simplicity of the instructions belies the effort required to increase your daily movement, get more sleep, or cut back on smoking. Whenever I focus my attention on doing more of something (sleep, movement) or less (spending money, caffeinating), friction materializes around that something, or at least it feels like that when I'm trying to implement lifestyle changes. For example, maybe there's an influx of invitations for socializing, some of which cost money that I'm trying not to spend. Adjustments to your way of living are not one-off decisions; they are things you will need to choose repeatedly over time and adapt to a variety of situations. Some lifestyle changes swiftly become the way you live now, and others will persistently feel like a lift.

One thing that does seem to help people commit is to have a clear understanding of the benefits. I'm going to make every effort not to offer advice on *how* to implement these changes, because the reality is that your considerations and circumstances are unique. Incremental changes (read: baby steps) do seem to stick better for most people—per the experts—and they also create opportunities to celebrate accomplishments. But this approach requires a realistic set of expectations around the timeframe or your progress. We tend to think of health as a binary thing—you're healthy or you're unhealthy—when in reality it's much more of a continuum that we are always shifting back and forth along over the course of our lives.

Movement (aka Exercise)

One thing that everyone in the medical community seems to be able to agree on is that moving our bodies is beneficial. There is also general consensus on the amount, frequency, and types of activities—150 minutes per week of moderate-intensity aerobic activity plus twice-weekly muscle-strengthening activity that works all major muscle groups (legs, hips, back, abdomen, chest, shoulders, and arms). This is not a realistic place to start for everyone and it's important to note that doing less than this is still beneficial to your overall health. There is evidence showing that moving our bodies helps to reduce stress and improve mood and leads to better long-term health outcomes and lower risk for cardiovascular disease, dementia, osteoporosis, and eight kinds of cancer (bladder, breast, colon, endometrium, esophagus, kidney, lung, and stomach)! There have even been small studies showing that strength training can help relieve hot flashes and night sweats. Movement has also been shown to help people with depression or anxiety and who have difficulty sleeping. In her book *The XX Brain,* Lisa Mosconi explains that, for women, lower intensity, higher frequency workouts are best for boosting metabolism and optimizing aerobic fitness.

Dr. Mosconi is aligned with health experts in encouraging you to incorporate physical movement into your days wherever possible— opting to walk instead of drive, or take the stairs instead of the elevator whenever possible. Yes, brisk walking counts as exercise. Seriously. Walking might be the most underutilized tool in the movement toolbox, and it makes exercise accessible to many people.

Strength training goes a long way to supporting your muscles, which, remember, are harder to maintain in the lead-up to and after menopause. You don't need a gym membership or even a home gym setup to get started. If you have a strip of floor somewhere that's the length of your body, you could begin with sit-ups, push-ups, and maybe some squats? Your entry point can be incredibly low-tech. Ease into things by starting with what you honestly believe you can do consistently. If you enjoy the activity you're doing, whether that's cycling, dancing, swimming, or walking, you are more likely to stick with it over time.

I'm a huge fan of micro goals—for example, walking for five minutes or doing the Scientific 7-Minute Workout (google it)— because it's so little time that it's hard to talk myself out of doing it. In fact, when I catch myself trying to weasel out of my activity, I often think, "If I had started moving when I started thinking, I would be four and a half minutes away from being done." As with all decision-making, you always have permission to change your mind about the kind of movement you do. Although culture has not conditioned you to think about it this way, an effective movement practice can be oriented around enjoyment.

Smoking and Your Body

There is never an easy time to quit smoking. The decision to consider breaking this habit is one that must be carefully considered in the scope of an individual's life. Like any serious change, not smoking will create friction both in your mind and in your world. I still think about a boss I had in my twenties who, after quitting, recounted the way that his activities had been measured in cigarettes and how disorienting it was to lose the activity that had served as the metronome of his daily life. Giving up things that you love or that make you feel comforted and relaxed is rough. There is plenty of change happening in the body during menopause, so adding quitting smoking to the list is a big ask. But the request, particularly when you are in the menopause transition, is warranted.

If you've been smoking for any length of time, I'm guessing that at least one person (a doctor, stranger, or loved one) has given you the rundown of health risks your behavior poses. The reason that people may bring the conversation up again when you begin transitioning to menopause is because of the impact the hormonal changes of menopause can have on aspects of your health that are also at an increased risk when you smoke.

Skin: Smoking reduces the amount of oxygen that reaches your skin, which is gradually becoming less resilient as estrogen declines, potentially giving you a yellow-gray complexion. Smoking during the reproductive years also leads to lower estrogen levels, which negatively impacts collagen and leads to more wrinkles.

Arteries/veins: Smoking thickens your blood, increases inflammation in the vessels, and increases the chances that clots could form and block the flow, plus it narrows your arteries, making you even more vulnerable to heart attacks and strokes at a time when declining estrogen is already impacting their flexibility. A woman who smokes is two to six times more likely to have a heart attack than one who doesn't. In studies of cisgender women, heart disease is the number one cause of death.

Bones: Smoking can make your bones more brittle, another risk factor that becomes even more serious when coupled with the effects of declining estrogen on your bones.

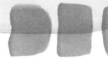

Food and Drink (aka Diet)

There are two ways that diet (what, how much, and when you eat and drink) intersects with menopause. The first is through the short (hot) list of individual foods and drinks that research has shown can exacerbate specific symptoms of peri and postmenopause. Caffeine, hot and spicy foods, and alcohol are all associated with increased hot flashes and night sweats. If you're seeking relief from those symptoms, it's worth tracking whether you experience them with increased frequency or intensity after you consume items on the hot list. In the event that you do notice a connection, that doesn't mean that you have to abstain from that food or drink item entirely (or forever).

Depending on the severity of your symptoms, it might make sense to take a week off from consuming things on the hot list and then experiment with adding them back in one at a time to see which ones affect your symptoms. You could also adjust the quantity you consume and see if that changes anything: do your hot flashes still flare if you dial back your caffeine intake or have half a glass of wine instead of a full one? Incremental adjustments require more patience, but they're also usually less disruptive to your routine and your emotions.

Changing anything about what or how you eat or drink can create friction in your life, even if it's only in the form of fielding questions from your friends, family, or coworkers about what you're eating or not eating. Maybe eating in a new way costs more money, doesn't taste as good, or means not participating in routine activities like a morning coffee ritual, having drinks at weekly happy hour with friends, or tasting every dish at a potluck dinner. Although I can't promise that they won't be awkward or challenging, these scenarios are navigable and, if you experience relief from your symptoms as a result, worth the trouble. As disappointing as it can be when you realize that something you enjoy is contributing to your bodily discomfort, understanding that relationship allows you to make informed decisions. Sometimes the enjoyment of items on the hot list is worth the disruption that comes with the symptoms they trigger, other times not so much, and you are the only person who can say what works best for you on a given day.

The second way that diet comes up in the menopause transition—weight management—is triggering in a totally different way. Like menopause, nutrition gets short shrift in the allopathic medical school curriculum. As we discussed at length in part two, medical professionals have long associated higher body weight with worse health outcomes, an association that has been questioned and scrutinized for decades. It's worth restating here that increasing your physical activity is more likely to positively impact your physical and emotional health than adjustments to your diet, because physical activity helps to prevent the loss of muscle mass and supports cardiovascular health.

There is a growing body of research to support a change in the current paradigm around weight and health outcomes, but changing our underlying ideas about body shape and size will take time and patience. Medical and cultural ideas about the body are intertwined, which makes everything surrounding one's diet high stakes in Western culture. Our physical shape and size are seen not only as reliable measures of our overall health, but also as representative of our value. Neither of those things is true, but that doesn't mean that they aren't real forces in our day-to-day lives.

As a result, changes in your body size are just as likely to inspire feelings within yourself as they are to elicit concerns from your

practitioner. The reality is that diet, nutrition, and weight are tough to confidently identify as causal to specific health conditions because there are so many factors at play in an individual person's life in addition to what and how they've been eating and drinking. In the interim, if your body gets bigger during menopause, you will probably receive recommendations to eat "healthier," exercise more, or reduce your caloric intake in order to make your body smaller. If you are interested in learning more about the movement and evidence for weight-neutral health care, please refer to the Health at Every Size website listed in the Resources section.

The sweet spot in terms of sating one's hunger, supplying the body with adequate energy and nutrients, and participating in social engagements that a person finds fulfilling is different for each individual. Finding your sweet spot requires a willingness to experiment and iterate, because your body's needs and desires will change throughout your life. If you do decide to implement dietary changes during your menopause transition, tread lightly. Changes to what and how you eat or drink always have the potential to lead to, or trigger former patterns of, disordered eating. Set yourself up to succeed by surrounding yourself with support, whether that means making sure you have time to prepare and cook meals or strategies for eating out with friends and family. In addition to making logistical arrangements, consider lining up emotional support from either a therapist or a supportive confidant in your life. Whether your body changes or you make changes to how you eat or drink, there's a high probability that you will have feelings about it, and it's nice to have a companion to help you navigate your emotions if things start to get weird.

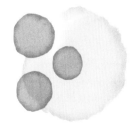

Alcohol and Your Body

Alcohol is generally hard on the body. It is disruptive to the brain, taxing to the heart, and creates extra work for the liver and pancreas. And yet alcohol is not only present at but woven directly into many of the social events we attend, like dinner parties, work happy hours, holidays, cookouts, and all manner of celebrations. The socially acceptable status of alcohol opens the door for habitual drinking without attracting concerns or negative attention. Whenever a doctor, any kind of doctor, asks me how many drinks I have in a week I give the same answer regardless of how true it is: seven. That number is sometimes true and sometimes not, but it is the number I think would be "okay" both in terms of my health and my identity. My response is more aspirational than factual.

At the onset of the COVID-19 pandemic, I regularly had at least two glasses of wine each night, often three, bringing my drink count up to more like 18 to 20 drinks a week. Here's the thing: it's not as if I didn't notice the effects. I was having daily headaches, disrupted sleep, and a general frustration that I felt like I didn't have full access to my brain, but drinking at the end of the day had stopped feeling like an option I was choosing; it became the default. Meanwhile, in my menopause research, I was learning about the additional labor already required by systems throughout our bodies to keep up with hormonal changes.

Because sex hormones do not decline along a gradual downslope, your body does a lot of work to keep your systems hovering around that stable midline that we call homeostasis. Liver function is particularly important for processing and moving excess estrogen out of the bloodstream and body to mitigate the effects of the peaks and subsequent plummeting. At the first whiff of toxin (alcohol in the blood), the liver drops everything and devotes itself to removing the toxin from the body, meaning that higher levels of estrogen are free to circulate throughout the body and impact tissues.

All of that being said, each individual body handles alcohol differently. Moderate alcohol consumption—one drink or fewer per day for women as defined by the Centers for Disease Control and Prevention—is associated

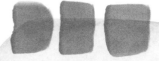

with both health risks and health benefits. Note that more than one drink each day does increase the risk of breast cancer. If you are experiencing night sweats or disrupted sleep, it might be worth taking a week or two off from drinking or to reduce your intake to one drink per day to see if your symptoms improve. If you struggle with chronic depression, consider that alcohol is a depressant. Per the CDC, one drink constitutes:

12 ounces of regular beer
(5 percent alcohol)

1.5 ounces of distilled spirit
(40 percent alcohol)

5 ounces of wine
(12 percent alcohol)

As discussed in the Food and Drink section, making changes to anything you consume as part of a social ritual can be challenging. The good news is that there's been tremendous growth in the non-alcoholic beverage category and lower alcohol or "session" cocktails making it increasingly possible to participate in cocktails or a round of beers without ingesting much (or any) alcohol. Even with these new options, there is the very real possibility that you will feel left out in the moment, watching others enjoy their drinks, and you may notice that changes in your behavior spark feelings in others too. Some folks may feel inspired to join you in making changes while others may feel that changes in your alcohol consumption are somehow passing judgment on their alcohol consumption. Because alcohol is so ingrained in a wide range of social and cultural events, it feels extra important to note that it's helpful to have a trusted friend or therapist at the ready to help you navigate a path with alcohol that supports your physical, social, and emotional needs (and process any fallout you encounter around changes in your intake) as you move through your transition.

Rest

Whether you are going through menopause during midlife or another time, everyone has many responsibilities at work, with their family, and/or in their community. Sleep quality can decline, meaning that you might wake up frequently as a result of disturbances like hot flashes or simply because you can't stop your mind from running through all that you need to do or from looping through your concerns. Interrupted sleep throughout the night can also be due to the complexity of hormonal changes that are occurring. Whether these disturbances wake you up in the middle of the night or not, you may find that you do not feel rested when you get up in the morning.

There is widespread agreement that sleep is important for our bodies, especially for our brains. The particulars, like how much sleep one needs, whether all kinds of sleep are equal, and when sleep should happen, are still being debated. The general guideline you're likely to hear from your practitioner is a minimum of seven to eight hours of sleep each night. If you are getting the recommended daily amount of sleep but you are not feeling rested when you wake up, it's worth talking about with your practitioner.

Sleep regulation is managed within the brain, and we know that fluctuating levels of estrogen and progesterone have an effect on the brain. Determining whether the cause of your sleep disruption is menopause, life circumstances, or a medical condition (hyperthyroidism, anxiety disorder, chronic pain) or is simply a result of aging is nearly impossible, but some of the symptoms of menopause—hot flashes, night sweats, anxiety, or depression—certainly can disrupt sleep.

There are a number of ways to improve your sleep hygiene, including things like sticking to a sleep schedule where you wake up and go to bed at the same time each day, keeping the room where you sleep cool and dark (or wearing a sleep mask), and using your bed only for sleeping and sex. In addition, consider trying no screen time an hour before bed, both because the blue light screens emit blocks melatonin (the hormone that makes you sleepy) and because the content (TV show, movie, internet, email) is stimulating. Think of sleep hygiene as training your body for regularly scheduled

sleep—teaching it how to wind down at the end of your day and how to soothe itself back to rest if you wake up before it's time to get up. These practices have proved helpful for many, but there are no guarantees that they will work for everyone who is in a position to implement them.

If you know that being awake in the middle of the night makes you panic, it might be worth trying a breathing practice (see the sidebar for an example) or finding a gentle activity to occupy your mind. I've had some luck with the one where you pick a letter in the alphabet and see how many words you can think of that start with that letter, but there are many others out there including counting sheep.

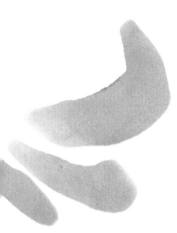

Breathing Yourself to Sleep

Deep breathing, sometimes called diaphragmatic breathing, stimulates the vagus nerve, part of your parasympathetic nervous system, lowering your body's stress response. It's hard to believe that something we do thoughtlessly every minute of every day of our lives could be so impactful, but breathing in a mindful way continues to show positive results in research studies. In addition to positive physiological effects, deep and slow breathing has an overall calming effect on the body including your heart rate, blood pressure, and muscles. Researchers have also observed that when participants in studies focus on breathing, they stop thinking about other things including problems or challenges that may be causing stress or anxiety.

Diaphragmatic breathing is one of the simplest breathing exercises you can do if you're struggling to sleep. Place one hand on your chest and the other on your diaphragm, the space right between the bottom of your ribs and your stomach. Inhale slowly and focus your attention on drawing air into your diaphragm so that the hand placed there will gently rise up while the hand on your chest remains relatively still. When you're ready to exhale, allow the air to slowly flow out of your diaphragm—you can purse your lips to make a whooshing sound like you might if you were blowing bubbles—and gradually draw your abdominal muscles inward as if you were softly squeezing the air all the way out.

I read (in a novel) about a phrase used to teach young children how to breathe slowly and deeply, and I've found that it helps to distract me with thoughts of pleasant things while also reminding me how to breathe deeply: *inhale to smell the flowers, exhale to blow out the birthday candles.*

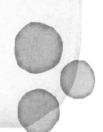

ADDITIONAL TREATMENT OPTIONS

Cognitive Behavioral Therapy

Cognitive behavioral therapy (CBT) focuses on shifting patterns of thinking to help individuals find better ways of coping with psychologically taxing situations. The goal in this type of therapy is to help you develop more effective ways of dealing with life and the stressors that you can't avoid. It has proved helpful with a few specific menopause symptoms like hot flashes and night sweats, insomnia, and even some anxiety and depression.

Talk Therapy

The transition to menopause can be an emotionally challenging time with unsettling feelings of anger or grief. Talking to a therapist can be a helpful practice for exploring, understanding, and potentially healing throughout the process. Whether your concerns are specific to the impacts of menopause on your daily life or more generally about what's happening in your life, having a safe space to talk about it on a regular basis can be a powerful source of support.

Acupuncture

An integral component of Traditional Chinese Medicine (TCM), acupuncture is an alternative medicine practice in which thin metal needles are inserted into the skin at specific points to support and improve the flow of qi, or the flow of energy throughout the body that TCM practitioners believe is responsible for overall health. Although there isn't data to support that acupuncture is an effective treatment for menopause symptoms, the National Institutes of Health has noted about a dozen ailments that can be effectively addressed with this therapy. Headaches, menstrual cramps, and fibromyalgia—all potential menopause symptoms—are included on that list. I spoke with people who have had great success managing their menopause symptoms with acupuncture in conjunction with a regimen of Chinese herbs prescribed by their TCM practitioner.

Bodywork

Whether you're seeking massage as a dedicated time to slow down, relax, and feel nurtured or chiropractic treatments to address specific pains or misalignments, bodywork can have positive effects on the body and mind. If you are experiencing joint pain or muscle stiffness or even having trouble getting comfortable enough to sleep, bodywork might provide some relief. Although there isn't research data pointing to bodywork as an effective intervention for specific menopause symptoms, some women report positive experiences with these treatments. Spending time with a practitioner who listens and addresses your needs can also do wonders in the midst of challenging symptoms or feelings.

"Sometimes I dance at home; that's actually my medicine for menopause right now, dancing at home. Lately it's 'Funky Cold Medina' . . . which is actually a song about Rohypnol, but it's really fun to dance to. If my energy gets too intense, or I'm transitioning and I'm getting that weird emotional-like lost space that happens more now, I just dance." —MAUDE

TOOLS FOR NAVIGATING CHANGE

One of the primary reasons that change is hard is that we live in culture that is neither accommodating nor forgiving. Organizational psychologist Adam Grant wrote, "You can't heal a sick culture with personal bandages," and though this is true, you do have agency in how you respond to challenging transitions. There are many frameworks out there for managing yourself and your feelings when the ground beneath your feet feels unsteady. The practices shared here are low-tech and accessible, which makes them easy to experiment with right away; there's no need to wait until you're in breakdown.

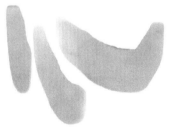

A Note about Taking Care of Yourself

Everything we've covered so far in this chapter is a way of taking care of yourself that requires or is based on clinical research and expertise. Professional stamps of approval are great, but they're not the qualifying bar we want to use for caretaking practices. If you didn't think you were going to have to explain or justify your choices to anyone, what would you opt to do (or not) as a means of taking care of yourself? Maybe it would be something like taking a walk, getting out into nature, getting a massage, or making yourself a tasty lunch, but it could just as easily be binge-watching your favorite show, taking a bath, enjoying a candy bar, or lying on the couch and absentmindedly flipping through magazines.

There are so many ways to tend to yourself. One of my favorite writers, Anne Lamott, swears by the healing powers of lotion massaged into her increasingly crepey skin. I know that I've found as much solace in organizing my closet as I have in a good night's sleep. Feeling cared for by oneself is a matter of personal preference. When you're at your breaking point, a caring act might simply be the one thing you can think to do or forget about doing that doesn't make you want to scream. Doing nothing can be as great a kindness to yourself as calling a friend who has a knack for lifting your spirits. It takes practice to take care of yourself, to learn to use your own experience to gauge what you need and then to give that thing to yourself or go and ask for it—so get your reps in, every chance you get.

F-Words

In her work coaching and counseling clients over the past decade-plus, somatic educator Jay Fields has observed that most of us respond to tough situations with one of three F-behaviors:

Figure it out: These folks believe that within each hardship is a code to be cracked and, if they could only figure it out, they could regain control of the situation.

Fix it: This crew sees discomfort as a problem to be solved, so they roll up their sleeves and get busy doing and iterating.

Fool yourself: These people are all about playing it cool, convincing themselves that it's no big deal and actually they don't care that much.

These are the things we see people do in movies, on TV, and in our day-to-day lives. We've watched these behaviors played out so many times that it seems like they are the only options, but they're not. Fields works with her clients to experiment with a fourth F-behavior:

Feel it: Feeling it means letting yourself feel the emotions or sensations in your body and acknowledging them by naming them.

It doesn't sound like much, but it's nothing short of astonishing what happens when you give yourself permission to *have* your experience instead of resisting it or trying to have an experience that you think would be more reasonable or appropriate, would make you look better, or would make things different.

All of the F-words "work" as tools for getting us through hard experiences, but those first three involve the extra effort required to operate on top of your feelings instead of allowing yourself to be fully who you are in the moment. Feeling your feelings doesn't mean you have to share them with others; it can be a completely private event. I've been known to whisper my feelings to myself in a bathroom stall at work. This can be as simple as saying the phrase, "I don't want to be feeling this feeling right now," or "This is exactly how I was afraid this would go, and I don't like it at all." If I'm in the midst of a challenging interaction, I might tell the other person that I need a minute to process what they're saying. Even if I can't physically walk away from them, if I can have a moment with no talking, I can use that quiet to release the pressure of big feelings that are begging for my attention and, likely, compromising my cognitive capacity.

Externalizing your feelings may not always be safe or even necessary, but ignoring them means that on some level you are leaving yourself hanging in a moment of distress. Big feelings are like a toddler who is really scared or excited and desperately needs to share their experience with another person. Even the most basic acknowledgment has the potential to help your feelings (or small child) to move through to a calmer place; if they're ignored, they are likely to misbehave or have a meltdown. It's hard to believe that we can offer this level of comfort to ourselves, especially when we're in emotional turmoil, but we absolutely can. We can also be soothed by interactions with others through an experience psychological experts call coregulation, where the sensitivity and engaged presence of another person can reduce our distress. A full exploration of self- and coregulation is beyond the scope of this book, but the emotional health books listed in the Resources section are good options for further exploration of these topics.

The fourth F-behavior—*feel it*—is a way of opening yourself up to your experience instead of resisting it. Emotions are like our immune system, offering us critical feedback about how our lives and the choices we're making are working (or not) for us. In periods of major transition, we can have "right," helpful feelings but on the "wrong" scale, like the emotional flashes one of my interviewees described as a defining experience of her menopause. When feelings seem too big for the situation, we get upset about being upset. The intensity of our feelings can be disorienting. Naming these feelings and talking about them, whether with ourselves in a caring way or with another person who cares about us, can go a long way toward right-sizing them.

A Name for Your Pain Is a Good Thing

Research has shown that giving a name to what we're feeling directly impacts our nervous system, dialing down the body's stress response. A few of the women I interviewed had developed vocabulary for experiences related to menopause symptoms. I've started calling the thing that happens when I lose the ability to focus "gnat mind," and I know someone else who calls it "brain weasels." Having a word for what I am experiencing helps me recognize when it is happening, which in turn helps me track it and notice if things change. It has also made it easier to talk about with my partner, friends, and even my therapist. Another serious benefit? Naming it something that makes me chuckle has made the whole thing a tiny bit less serious.

Slowing Your Roll

It's impossible to talk about slowing down or resting without acknowledging that doing either requires some degree of privilege. Every time I hear or read a practitioner tell people to work less, sleep more, and take better care of themselves during their menopause transition, there's a part of my brain that throws its hands up in the air and says, *Do you know anything about the world we're living in?* And yet, I agree that all those recommendations can positively impact overall health. It's an unfortunate reality that, even for individuals in dire need, a full-blown downshift to rest and recuperation is often not feasible, so slowing down will need to be an incremental practice for most of us until we see massive structural change in our economic systems and cultural beliefs around productivity. Tending to your life in the modern world is like a high-wire act where you are forever balancing between the dueling realities of *life is precious* and *I live in the world*. In an attempt to honor that both of these realities are true, we're going to explore a couple of micro-adjustments that have the potential to create a bit of breathing room in your life.

"I have had a major surgery that literally sent me into a full-blown menopause, so my body deserves to realign itself. My body deserves to have the opportunity naturally without emotional weightedness that I could put on it. My body deserves to go through its natural state and to heal itself. I just want to give my body a chance to reconcile itself with itself in this new space that I'm in." —ALATHEA

Let's begin with three revolutionary words: *not right now*. When someone asks for your time, energy, or attention, you have the option to say no. If that doesn't feel like a real option, or you need some time to build up the courage to say no, these three words make a wonderful baby step. They are like the softest wedge between your needs and the press of the world's demands. If you don't believe me, try it the next time someone asks you for help while you're in the middle of something (even if that something is just you taking a walk for no reason or watching a mediocre show). Tell them, "Yes. Absolutely I will help you. Happy to do it, just not right now." From there, the two of you can figure out a time that honors their needs and yours.

One reason that slowing down is difficult is because we fear that we won't ever speed up again. It's a valid concern, because sometimes when we slow down, we realize that we like our new pace, and we genuinely don't want to speed back up. Other times the reality is that we cannot do things in the exact same way we did before. In situations where slowing down feels scary because it looks like poorly disguised giving up, developing a more nuanced vocabulary for slowing down can help. What if, instead of saying that you're going to slow down, you add some specificity to it, maybe a plan to *set something down for a week or a month* and to then check in with yourself to see if you want to pick it back up. Or, does it make sense to tell yourself that you're pressing the pause button and giving yourself permission to unpause at the end of the day, or the season? Whatever language feels kind and gentle can work here, especially when paired with calendar reminders or pinky swears with that dear friend who doesn't let you off the hook when it counts.

If both of these seem like silly little verbal tricks, it's because they are—you're onto me. The thing is, the way we say stuff makes a difference. This is why we get stopped in our tracks when someone asks us if we would talk to a beloved friend or family member the way we talk to ourselves. Find the words that feel right to you, say them with love and tenderness, and don't rush it. My sister, who has been teaching elementary school for decades, has one of the most generous and true responses when she spots distress in her students.

She sidles up next to them, eyes trained in the same direction as theirs, and gently reminds them, "It won't always be like this." When she says it to me, sometimes it helps and sometimes it makes me want to give her a hard shove, but what I appreciate about it is the way it offers a bit of comfort without a specific timeline or the expectation that I will start to feel different in the moment. Instead, it creates a little bit of space for me to catch my breath where I am, and a reminder that I don't have to leave before I'm ready nor stay there forever.

7

GETTING SUPPORT

The biggest learning from my conversations with people in the midst of or on the other side of their menopause transition was this: their ability to navigate the experience was defined less by the symptoms and emotions they encountered than by how well resourced they were. Resourced here doesn't mean that they had money, though that is helpful; it's about having a network of people in your life who keep you feeling connected and supported through the ups and downs—the folks who are committed to being there for you even when they don't understand exactly what you're going through.

It's the partner who hears you out about not feeling your sexiest. Instead of insisting that you are, they tell you that, although that's not their experience of you, they can imagine how crummy seeing yourself that way must feel, and they ask what, if anything, they can do to support you. It's the group of friends you do happy hour with each week who hear that you're taking a break from alcohol and do a little legwork to find bars and restaurants with great nonalcoholic cocktails, making sure you will have choices that are more fun than a fizzy water. It's the doctor who makes you feel accompanied in subtle ways like saying *we* when they talk about your treatment options, "*We* are going to figure out how to get you some relief from your symptoms. Let me just run through what I heard when you described what's going on so *we* know that *we're* not missing anything." In short, these are the people who thoughtfully consider you and your needs, the people who make space for your experience.

"My husband, I'm almost in tears when I think about the level of support that this man has given as a friend. And we don't talk about menopause like every day—probably I talked about it more with you than him—but just the level of support that he's given me to just be. To just be me, and to understand what that looks like and what it is in this season of my life." —ALATHEA

The kind of community support you need during menopause looks a lot like the kind that would support you in everyday life, with a couple of important additions like buddies you can talk with openly about body stuff and also maybe some medical expertise. If you are in a situation where you feel that your network is strong (yay!), you might be looking for ideas about how to ask your wonderful web of people for help. We're going to review menopause-specific resources you might need, ways of asking the people in your life for the kind of support you need during your transition, and how to talk about menopause with others.

WHEN YOU NEED A MEDICAL PROFESSIONAL

There are so many reasons why you see the kind of medical professional you do. Money, insurance (or lack of it), transportation, availability, beliefs, a need for specialized training or expertise, and recommendations or referrals can all be factors in determining how you end up sitting in one waiting room instead of another. As we've discussed, the field of medicine has room for many perspectives. Regardless of your age when you begin experiencing perimenopause symptoms, you've probably picked a lane—allopathic, naturopathic, Traditional Chinese Medicine, or another modality—where you are most comfortable, within the bounds of your insurance, or a place you can reliably afford and access care. Menopause is not a reason to change lanes, but it could be helpful to seek out a practitioner within your lane who has experience with (and an interest in) patients going through menopause.

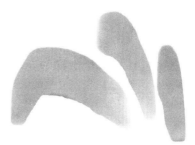

What's a Menopause Specialist?

As previously discussed, menopause does not get in-depth coverage in medical school programs. Even the specialists we imagine would have learned the most about women's health—obstetricians and gynecologists—do not focus much time and attention on this stage of our reproductive trajectory. There is no menopause specialist designation within the American Board of Medical Specialties, so the only way to know whether or not your current practitioner is an informed resource for you during and after your transition is to ask them about their clinical experience. The North American Menopause Society (NAMS), a nonprofit devoted to the health of women in menopause, offers a training and certification that covers the broad range of menopause experiences and health considerations. You can tell if a doctor has this certification by looking for the letters NCMP (NAMS Certified Menopause Practitioner) as part of their credentials. NAMS also maintains a searchable roster of certified practitioners. If your current practitioner does not have the certification, it doesn't mean that they cannot help you or that they don't know about menopause, but it does mean that you'll want to ask them some questions to understand their level of experience and protocols for working with patients throughout their transition.

VETTING PRACTITIONERS

Every individual on the planet deserves to have a practitioner who is a true partner in their health. The realities of our healthcare system are such that access to and quality of time with practitioners is not equitable.

Whether you are in a position where you have the time, money, and motivation to seek specialized menopause expertise or you simply want to understand your current practitioner's experience, these questions and considerations regarding potential answers will help you to gather information.

Q: How much experience do you have working with patients or clients who are going through the transition to menopause?

A: If they say they have a lot of experience, you might also ask them to describe their approach or philosophy about menopause, or how they work with their patients throughout the transition. If they say they have some experience, it's worth asking them about their comfort level in treating someone going through menopause. If they tell you that menopause is a natural process that all women go through and that it's just something that people need to endure, you might want to ask around among your friends to see if anyone has a practitioner with a more nuanced perspective on the transition. You might not ever need or want specialized care, but if you begin to experience challenging symptoms, you'll be glad to have referrals for practitioners who are more deeply engaged in menopause care.

Q: Can you walk me through the long-term health considerations I should be aware of for people my age who are approaching, in the midst of, or on the other side of the menopause transition?

A: Answers to this question will vary, as they should, depending on your specific situation. If you're twenty-eight and about to enter surgical menopause, the considerations will be different from those of a forty-seven-year-old who is just beginning to notice irregular menstrual cycles and wondering if she's entering perimenopause. Even if you're not looking for symptom relief at the time you ask this question, the thoughtfulness of their answer—Does it consider your health history? Does it take your concern seriously?—can offer you a sense of their process with their patients.

Q: Are there any treatment modalities or options for menopause-related symptoms that you have strong feelings about (either in favor of or opposed to)?

A: As they respond, listen for any strong opinions or statements about any category of treatment—pharmaceuticals, nonpharmaceuticals, bodywork—that don't feel open for discussion or for consideration of your perspective or experiences. Also be on the lookout for rigid ideas about what "healthy" looks like. If you do hear something that doesn't land well with you, that might be a time to ask the practitioner to unpack their thinking or tell you more about it.

NAVIGATING APPOINTMENTS

Knowing that practitioners are working with time constraints, it can be difficult to ask them to slow down or unpack their expertise in greater detail for you. If you get turned around because of the information they share or because they continue to rush, you might ask them if there is a way for you to get follow-up questions answered. Remind them that the terminology and information they're sharing is new to you (maybe it's even the first time you've heard it), and that you need some time to take it in before you know the questions you want to ask.

Here are some questions and prompts that may help you advocate for yourself in the moment or, at the very least, better understand your specific physiology and your practitioner's recommendations. I'm in favor of taking a notebook into my appointments because it helps me remember my questions and also take notes on their responses. You could also consider recording your appointment on a smartphone or other device, with the consent of the practitioner.

1. Can you talk me through how you got to that assessment (prescription, lifestyle change, or any other recommendation)? I feel like it might help me to understand what you see in my condition, symptoms, or health history that makes this course of action seem like the best next step.

2. I'm not sure that I got that—and this is really important to me. Can you talk me through it one more time?

3. This is a new experience for me in my body, and while I understand that it's not life-threatening or an illness, it is significantly impacting my life (be as specific as you can about how). Can you help me understand treatment options?

4. What is the goal with this treatment, and how are we going to assess that it's working? Can you walk me through the plan?

5. I've got some budget constraints that I'd like to share so that you understand what options might work better for me.

6. Is this treatment option compensating for something that I could accomplish in other ways that might not involve purchasing a prescription or over-the-counter product?

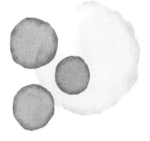

IT'S AMAZING WHAT YOU CAN'T DO YOURSELF

Years ago, I had a counselor who had a knack for asking questions that helped me understand that some of the stumbling blocks I kept tripping over were, in fact, my own subconscious beliefs. For example, when I casually mentioned that I liked to do things on my own, she asked me what I thought about people who asked for help. I'm not sure how it's possible to have no idea that you have certain ideas, but I just know it is the case, because that afternoon I discovered that I had some pretty garbage-y opinions about people who ask for help (they're disorganized, less competent, unprepared, inconsiderate, flaky). Rationally, I knew that we all need help sometimes, and yet I had this deep-seated belief that if you were in a position of needing help it was because you were doing something wrong.

Our culture still swings around the maypole of rugged individualism; it just gets dressed up in new clothes for each generation. For example, the era of self-empowerment ushered in by white feminists in the late twentieth century paved the way for the #girlboss of today; the underlying message to women being that we can do and have it all, but only if we are willing to work and believe hard enough. If you fail, that's on you. We never really moved beyond this pull-yourself-up-by-your-bootstraps mentality. Even the seemingly positive ideas of self-empowerment and self-care are often used as ways of saying *you should be able to take care of yourself, so why are you asking for help?* What's consistently left out is the baseline support that every individual needs to effectively care for themselves. In other words, you can't pull yourself up with bootstraps you don't have or achieve equity through self-empowerment when the structures you live within systemically disempower you.

Menopause is a terrible time to dig in your heels about doing it all by yourself, because even though it might not be visible to you or to anyone else, your body is doing extra work trying to keep up with the shifting sands of your hormones. Erratic body temperatures, shitty

sleep, and an itchy vagina are just a few of the reasons you might not be feeling on top of your game. If you don't think now is the time to ask for help, then I might ask, when? As a person who is conditioned to reflexively answer no when someone asks if I need help, I can attest to the unlearning that has to happen in order for me to sense the internal signals letting me know when it's time to raise my hand and say yes instead. It takes practice. You don't have to start with asking someone to help you to decide whether to leave your current relationship; maybe start with some small stuff. Let the bagger carry your groceries to the car, say yes when someone offers you a glass of water or a ride when you actually need one, or ask a friend if they'll make you dinner at the end of your busiest day next week.

I want to be very clear that you're not always going to like the help that you get. You can find the help of others distasteful for a whole host of reasons, including that it's more than you asked for, it's not enough, the person helping needs too much appreciation, the help doesn't come when you need it, or it's just straight-up the wrong kind. Help will not disappear your struggles, but it is still a marked improvement over trying to manage everything on your own. Yes, you will open yourself up for potential disappointment, but you also won't be alone anymore in that place in your mind where your fears and troubles can be so big and monstrous.

WHAT DO YOU NEED?

This question doesn't seem like it would be hard to answer, but sometimes it is because it's not always obvious exactly what the problem you're facing is when you're in the midst of a struggle. In moments where I feel overwhelmed, I default to thinking that I need practical assistance like someone to help me move heavy stuff, or chop a lot of things up, or pick me up thirty minutes later than we planned. Sometimes that is exactly what I need just because I'm in a pinch, but other times what I need is a safe space to vent. Learning to tell the difference between those moments helps you figure out who to ask and what exactly you're asking of them.

There are situations where you don't have the capacity to think about what you need, and you have to rely on the people around you to assess what's happening and check in with you about what's working and what's not. Menopause can be a bit like this at times because it's new and evolving for you and everybody around you. In addition to physical changes you experience, you might have an emotional response to those changes. If it's possible in the moment to pause and ask yourself, *Am I uncomfortable, am I upset, or both?* your response can guide you in asking for the support you need. There is also nothing wrong with saying, *I don't know exactly what I need right now, I just know that I'm not feeling okay. Can we talk it through together?*

A close friend called me from the airport in a panic. She was on her way to her in-laws for a long weekend and feeling overwhelmed by the recent onslaught of perimenopause symptoms—sleeplessness, vasomotor instability, and mood swings. Together, we started unpacking the potential sources of her distress. It was clear that she wasn't concerned that her in-laws wouldn't understand or accommodate her needs, so I asked her if she was embarrassed about what her body was doing. She said no, but what she said right after that was definitely something that can get in the way of us seeking help when we need it.

The thought of being the center of attention, because of her need for specific accommodations, was making her uncomfortable—squirmy, in fact. She didn't want her perimenopause symptoms to be the only thing her in-laws saw when they looked at her, or for that part of her to be the central focus of the visit. That's when I understood that the root of her panic was about the visit and also about something much bigger than the visit. She felt like she was backed into a corner where she only had two crappy options to choose from: get her needs met but risk people she cares about perceiving her differently or suffer in secret. First, we acknowledged together how scary it is to feel like you don't have control over your body, especially around other people. And then we talked about a third option, where she would ask for what she needed and also tell her in-laws that these changes in her body were still new for her, that she was finding her way through them, and what worked best for her was others trusting that she would ask for help when she needed it.

WHO CAN YOU ASK?

Knowing what kind of help you need can guide how (and who) you ask for support. Here are some examples of various types of help and support you may need throughout your menopause transition and suggestions of how you might ask for them.

Even though I believe wholeheartedly in the power of having another person witness my struggles, I'm not always ready to show the gnarliest parts of myself to anyone else. If you don't think you can say your worst thoughts or biggest fears aloud to another human being yet, try shouting them at your car radio or into your pillow. I've also whispered a few in the shower and imagined them flowing right down the drain. The idea is to release the pressure that's built up inside you gradually, like the release valve on a pressure cooker, allowing all of that steam a graceful way to exit so it doesn't hurt anyone (including you).

Advice/insights: When you're seeking sage advice or insights on how to solve a problem, look for that person in your network who has navigated a similar situation or a person whose way of being you admire. You don't have to ask this person to tell you what you should do, though you can. You could say something like, "Hey, I'm struggling a bit with this situation, and I'm wondering if I could tell you about it and you could tell me how you might approach it or think about it. I've always admired how you think about things, and I wonder if hearing your thought process might give me some new ideas."

Logistical support: Moving, lifting, and accommodating everything from your schedule to your physical comfort, or energy level—all of these are examples of tactical help you can request from other people. Think about who you know who has offered to help you in the past or look for someone who seems well positioned to help you with little effort. For example, if you want a ride to school for your child while your car is in the shop, maybe you know another parent who lives nearby and has room in their car? One of the reasons people hesitate before agreeing to help people with logistical stuff is that they worry that if they do it once they'll be on the hook to do it forever. Taking a beat to think realistically about how much help you need and for how long and then being clear about those parameters when you make your request can create some natural boundaries for you and the other person. Let's say you want to ask a coworker to support you in adjusting your schedule so you can make it to a recurring doctor's appointment. "I'd like to shift our meeting to 3 p.m. indefinitely. I'm flexible on the day of the week, but really need it to start at 3 p.m. so we can finish reliably by 4:30 p.m."

Listening: If you're in that zone where you want to kick anyone who glibly offers you solutions to your problem or you are totally twisted up in your own situation, it might help to ask someone if they can hear you out without weighing in. There are so many brilliant tactical minds out there, conditioned to serve the world by offering solutions to every problem they encounter, but maybe what you're looking for is that person who has a knack for making you feel accompanied in the struggle and that the way that you are, even at your worst and whiniest, is okay. And all you might need to say to them is, "Can I just vent for a minute?" Once you've said your piece it's up to you if you want to follow it up with something like, "You know, I feel like I'm spinning on this topic, can you tell me what you heard in what I just shared?" You might be surprised what you're able to hear in your own words when they come out of someone else's mouth.

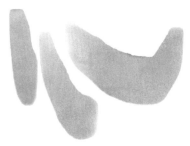

WHAT CAN YOU DO ABOUT IT?

> "I would call my mom and dad, my husband, my sisters, because I knew what those conversations would sound like and feel like. I knew that I would get encouragement, but I would also not get babying. I would get consoling and comforting, but at the same time, the conversation won't let you linger in self-pity." —ALATHEA

THE UNHELPABLE PLACE

The first time I remember being in the unhelpable place was in junior high, standing at the mouth of my bedroom closet before school trying to figure out what to wear. That is where I would cower, in the depths of emotional collapse, while my older sister tried to convince me that I looked great in each of the rejected outfits lumped in soft mounds around my feet. Blasted with fear and self-loathing, all I could hear in her enthusiastic endorsements was this: there isn't a problem here, and the way that you're feeling is wrong. Humiliation washed over me, and things began to feel absolutely desperate. I know now that she was doing her best, and I wish I could say that I responded with grace, but I didn't. I went with the cornered-animal strategy of vicious defensiveness because it was the only way I knew to help me feel a little bit safer.

Shame about how I treated my sister on those mornings followed me around for years, as did a concern about the monster within me that had the potential to emerge and lash out whenever I landed in an unhelpable place. I hated the way that this fear of myself

made me petulant, as if other people had to handle me with kid gloves. What I've come to understand about the unhelpable place is that it's a situation where I'm fighting the pressure to feel better or different about something before I actually do. It's not exactly true that I cannot be helped, it's that the help I need is not the kind that's offered most frequently—the kind that requires me to feel some other way—usually *better*—than I do, or to move through my emotions at someone else's pace.

Recalling those painful moments, standing in front of my closet in total breakdown, I can see that what might have truly helped me was for someone to acknowledge what I was feeling without trying to change it. In short, I wanted someone to make me feel like I wasn't crazy for feeling the way that I did. These days I am thoughtful about how and who I ask for help, and my spidey-sense is better at letting me know when a situation is particularly "hot" for me. Giving a name to the unhelpable place helped me to now recognize it when it's happening and prompts me to tell the other person, "I'm aware that I'm telling myself a story that the way that I'm feeling right now is making you impatient with me." Or to say explicitly that what I need in the moment is for it to be okay that I'm not feeling okay about the matter at hand.

THANK YOU, BUT NO THANK YOU

Help and advice can shift a stuck situation, but they can also just plain piss you off. When you ask for support and what comes your way isn't working, speaking up about that can make you feel like an ingrate. When things go sideways you have the option to speak up or stick it out. Either way you might offend someone or end up feeling worse off than before. If you do want to speak up and are struggling to find the words, here are a few gentle ideas to get you started.

> **SITUATION:** You asked for help and someone started helping you, but it's not working and you're not sure why.

> **RESPONSE:** Hey, can we stop for a second. Thank you for your willingness to get in here with me and help. As we're going

through this, I'm realizing that I might need a bit more time to think about what I actually need. I thought this was the right thing, but I'm feeling a bit overwhelmed/agitated/frustrated, and I don't want to take that out on you. Can I let you know if and when I'm ready to try again?

Shortcut: You know, I thought I was ready for help, and I'm not. Can I take some time and let you know if and when I am ready?

SITUATION: You didn't ask for help, but you're getting it and you want it to stop.

RESPONSE: This is a difficult thing to say because I can see how much you want to help me with/through this, but I'm not feeling open to it right now. I'll let you know if I want to talk about this at some point.

If you genuinely appreciate that they tried, you could also thank them for reaching out.

SITUATION: You asked for someone to listen, but they are disagreeing with you, or offering solutions or words of encouragement, and it's not working for you.

RESPONSE: I appreciate that it might be uncomfortable for you to hear about some of the challenging feelings I'm experiencing. I'm not saying that these things are the truth, but they are how I'm feeling right now.

A bit more of a flex: Can you see how I might feel like you're saying that what I'm feeling isn't okay or isn't real?

TALKING IT OUT

It's not always comfortable to talk about your body, especially parts of your body that have been labeled *private*. Even if no one explicitly told you to keep quiet about the components of your reproductive system and anything related to them, you probably noticed the way people lower their voices, use slang, and speak in metaphor when talking about their vulvas, vaginas, and menstruation, let alone sex. In addition, disagreement about how to discuss, manage, and feel about menopause stems from some of our core cultural conflicts around what it means to live in a gendered body. Like so many other aspects of women's health, menopause feels polarized; it's paradoxically overhyped and actively dismissed. Nearly every woman I spoke with throughout the duration of my research and writing said something like, *It's just that no one is talking about this,* or *Why aren't we talking about this?* Here's the good and bad news all in one: this will not change unless we start talking about it.

So, let's look at some ways that you can begin to do that in a way that makes sense for you.

> "It's something that I have said to people out loud: *Why did no one talk to me about this? Why did no one have this conversation with me about what this could be like?* Unless we have a really good supportive friend or family unit or group, we're not super encouraged to talk about these kinds of things. And if we are, it's to be ashamed of them, or make them stop, or fix them." —AIMEE

"I have had to practice making it something that I am not embarrassed to talk about because one of the things I'm trying to do from a personal and political perspective is to normalize it more. A friend that I've had for a long time stood in my kitchen one day and told me about her hysterectomy and said, 'I think that women have to talk to each other about this stuff.' It really stuck in my mind, so I try to remember when I'm with my women friends and something like this comes up, to talk about my own experience in a really frank way." —MELISSA

TALKING AMONGST OURSELVES

Talking to each other before, during, and after menopause is a valuable means of sharing information that can help us understand what's happening and hear about a variety of ways to navigate a range of experiences and the emotions that accompany them. If you did not grow up talking to family members, friends, or really anyone about your body, this is probably going to feel awkward at first. I know that my tendency is to reach for a book or do some internet sleuthing before calling a friend to talk about vaginal discomfort, changes in my menstrual bleeding, or anything related to sex. Books and the internet are great sources of information, and they're also ways of keeping my body private in a way that, for me, is also grounded in a fear that my body is gross or wrong somehow. That isn't the reason for every person's discretion, so it's important to respect each individual person's choices about engaging in explicit conversations about the body.

The menopause experience is not a monolith. Carrying into your conversations the awareness that menopause is both a real and far-reaching set of physiological changes in the body and a collection of cultural constructs is one way to create a more flexible space for people to ask questions and share their experiences. Here are some prompts and notes to support you in having conversations about menopause with a range of people in your life and in your community.

"I definitely know when we keep things inside, we don't realize that where we are and what we may be experiencing is also being experienced by millions of others. I hate to say misery loves company, but I think misery loves to know that it's not by itself. So, for women who are in this season who are being demeaned, devalued, [and told] *get over it, it couldn't be that bad,* my heart is heavy for that, because she gets to be vulnerable and she needs to be fragile. Not to drown in that fragility, but she should have community, and if we don't have it from our spouses and our kids, are we able to trust each other? To lean into each other?" —ALATHEA

When You Just Want to Talk about All of It!

Because we're so used to people not talking about menopause, it's easy to overthink the questions you need to get a conversation going. Keep it as simple as you can so the person responding can feel free to talk about the parts of their experience that they feel most compelled to share.

What's it like? It's amazing how far this question can take you in conversation with another person (or a group of people). Seriously, if you gathered up three friends and started by having each person answer this question at whatever level they choose, you might not even need another question. This is an open question that allows the person responding to disclose the parts of their experience that feel salient, and to talk about menopause in their terms. Listeners can both glean insights about physiology and emotions and access new language to describe their own experiences.

What, if anything, made you feel supported? This is another invitation for people to consider where they have support in their lives as they go through this transition. Sometimes it's helpful to hear others talk about accepting help and support, especially if they are people whom you love and admire, because it reminds you that it is totally okay and normal to not be able to do everything on your own.

When You Have Questions about Specific Symptoms or Treatments

Do you have any experience with [*fill in the blank*]? Do you know much about [*fill in the blank*]? For example: *hormonal migraines, vaginal dryness, taking black cohosh.* If they say no, you could ask if they know anyone who does. In addition, remember that everyone's body is different, so try to keep your expectations in check about tips, tricks, and treatments that worked wonders for other people. That said, if something is working for you, there's no reason to keep it a secret!

I read/heard about this treatment for [*fill in the blank*] and it sounds interesting, but I wonder if I'm missing something? This is a great way to ask about things that sound too good to be true.

When You're Listening to Someone Share Information That You Think Is Incorrect

I haven't heard that before—tell me more? This question allows the other person to share more information rather than defend a position. It's possible that you misunderstood what they were originally saying; this allows you to learn more. And it creates more of an opening for you to ask additional, clarifying questions. The fact that menopause is different for everyone and that medical professionals don't see eye to eye about the best way to address it means that we can expect plenty of conflicting information. Also, remember that there are different ideologies at play about the body, women, and aging (not to mention that we're still living in times of truthiness).

Online or In-Person?

No right or wrong answer here. Both online and in-person interactions have the potential for connection and an exchange of useful information, which is ultimately what you're after. If you are going through the menopause transition at a different time than your peers, you may find yourself seeking other avenues for conversation, like a support group or an online group of people in a similar situation. There are volumes of stories about people living with symptoms and conditions at the edge of medical knowledge who have found online communities to be crucial sources of validation and information about courses of treatment, diagnosis, and research. Finding a space where you can feel seen and heard is what matters most. You probably have a sense of what form and format works best for you; start there.

TALKING TO PEOPLE WHO WON'T EXPERIENCE MENOPAUSE

There is no requirement that you tell anyone about your experience with menopause. You can go through your transition, maybe (or maybe not) talking to your friends online or in-person about your shared experience, and come out the other side without having described what it was or wasn't to anyone else. And, there may be people (family, friends) whom you want to understand what's happening in your life. Depending on what kinds of conversations you have with these people about changes in your body, it could be intimidating or no big deal. The brief outline here is meant to support you, should you have the urge to share your menopause experience with someone who will not personally ever experience it—or even someone who will, but not for many years.

Some version of this script might also work for you if someone asks you about your menopause experience. When people are curious, it's always a good idea to ask them what it is they want to know before you dive in, because they might literally just want to know what it is, or instead they could be truly wondering about what you're going through. Feel free to dabble in metaphor, but avoid giving reproductive organs nicknames, which can create a sense that their proper names are too embarrassing to say aloud. You don't have to provide a detailed history lesson on women's health or a roster of the cultural constructs at play, but it might be helpful to note that ideas about menopause are informed by all of these things plus an individual's lived experiences. If they seem to want more information than you have, go ahead and refer them to resources that were helpful to you. And, of course, if the question coming at you feels unfriendly, you can always respond with a question of your own, like, *Why do you ask?*

The statements offered here are a starting place; not all of them will resonate with you, and they certainly will not cover everything you might want to discuss. Take the time to make them yours. And then practice, especially if these topics and combinations of words are not things you're used to saying out loud. Hearing them in your voice a few times can be a way of clarifying what's more important for you to communicate and building the confidence that you can speak them aloud.

Can We Talk?

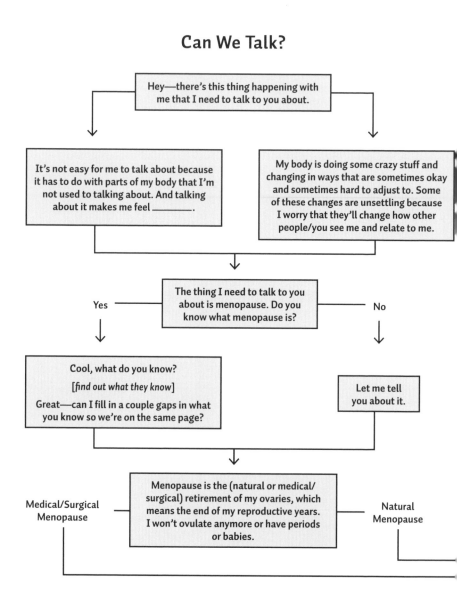

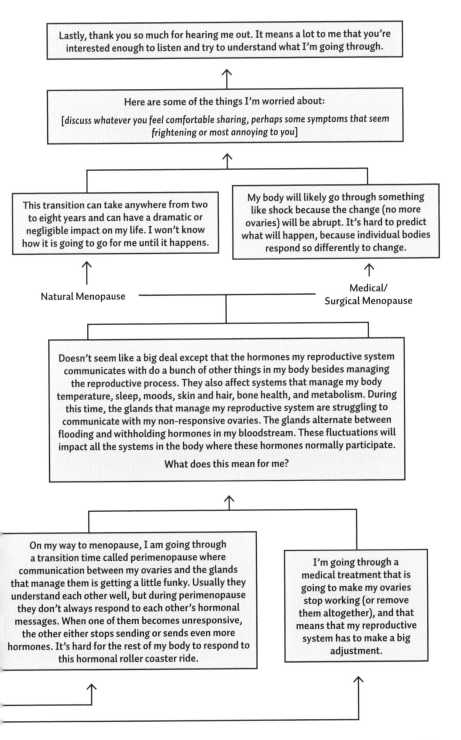

Lastly, thank you so much for hearing me out. It means a lot to me that you're interested enough to listen and try to understand what I'm going through.

Here are some of the things I'm worried about:

[discuss whatever you feel comfortable sharing, perhaps some symptoms that seem frightening or most annoying to you]

This transition can take anywhere from two to eight years and can have a dramatic or negligible impact on my life. I won't know how it is going to go for me until it happens.

My body will likely go through something like shock because the change (no more ovaries) will be abrupt. It's hard to predict what will happen, because individual bodies respond so differently to change.

Natural Menopause — Medical/ Surgical Menopause

Doesn't seem like a big deal except that the hormones my reproductive system communicates with do a bunch of other things in my body besides managing the reproductive process. They also affect systems that manage my body temperature, sleep, moods, skin and hair, bone health, and metabolism. During this time, the glands that manage my reproductive system are struggling to communicate with my non-responsive ovaries. The glands alternate between flooding and withholding hormones in my bloodstream. These fluctuations will impact all the systems in the body where these hormones normally participate.

What does this mean for me?

On my way to menopause, I am going through a transition time called perimenopause where communication between my ovaries and the glands that manage them is getting a little funky. Usually they understand each other well, but during perimenopause they don't always respond to each other's hormonal messages. When one of them becomes unresponsive, the other either stops sending or sends even more hormones. It's hard for the rest of my body to respond to this hormonal roller coaster ride.

I'm going through a medical treatment that is going to make my ovaries stop working (or remove them altogether), and that means that my reproductive system has to make a big adjustment.

ACKNOWLEDGMENTS

While authoring a companion for the many people who will experience menopause, I required the professional and friendly companionship of many people. I'd like to thank a few of them here.

First and foremost, a heartfelt thank-you to all the individuals who spoke with me, formally and informally, about your experiences of menopause. Your words illuminate the multifaceted nature of menopause, and they offer a reminder of the potential that shared stories have to make menopause less mysterious. Special thanks to the two friends whose openness about their symptoms and sentiments years ago inspired me to learn all that I could about menopause and share it widely.

I am deeply grateful to my coauthor, Dr. Tori Hudson; I could not have created this unique guide without you. Your passion for women's health and for all people who experience menopause was evident in the many hours you spent patiently answering my questions. Thank you for your enduring candor and good humor. Big thanks to the team at Roost Books for engaging thoughtfully and enthusiastically with this topic and me. Special thanks to Audra Figgins for her swift and supportive editing. And much gratitude to Juree Sondker for seeing an opening in the menopause space and inviting me into this project.

Camilla and Matt Pettle, Norma Steiner, Lola Millholland, Annie Moss, Jennifer Koo, Bernardo Rodriguez, Rachel Rockey, Joe Paganelli, Shawn Westfall, and Wendy Noonan, thank you all for accompanying me in a variety of ways—on phone, on foot, and in friendship—as I wandered through the themes of this project and the process of writing it. An extra special thank-you to Wendy for your work as a thoughtful early reader and editor. You have a knack for helping me understand what I'm trying to say (and how to say it better).

Jay Fields, thank you for sharing your brain, heart, and communication skills with this project and me; we are both greatly improved as a result of your generosity. Nancy Nowacek, this book would not exist if you hadn't fueled the initial spark years ago that led to our humble, self-published booklet about menopause. Thank you for your relentless encouragement; I would not have done this and many other wonderful things without it.

Last and in no way least, thank you, Michael Claypool, for making space for me to be me, both within our shared life and out in the world.

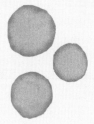

RESOURCES

MENOPAUSE

Before Your Time: The Early Menopause Survival Guide by Evelina
   Weidman Sterling
Hot and Bothered: Women, Medicine, and Menopause in Modern America
   by Judith A. Houck
Hot Flashes: Women Writers on the Change of Life edited by
   Lynne Taetzsch
The Menopause: A Comic Treatment edited by MK Czerwiec
Menopause Manifesto: Own Your Health with Facts and Feminism by
   Dr. Jen Gunter
*The Slow Moon Climbs: The Science, History, and Meaning of
   Menopause* by Susan P. Mattern

WOMEN'S HEALTH

Belabored: A Vindication of the Rights of Pregnant Women by Lyz Lenz
*Come As You Are (Revised and Updated): The Surprising New Science That
   Will Transform Your Sex Life* by Emily Nagoski
Everything below the Waist: Why Health Care Needs a Feminist Revolution
   by Jennifer Block
Fearing the Black Body: The Racial Origins of Fat Phobia by
   Sabrina Strings
The Fifth Vital Sign: Master Your Cycles and Optimize Your Fertility by Lisa
   Hendrickson-Jack
*Hormone Repair Manual: Every Woman's Guide to Healthy Hormones after
   40* by Lara Briden, ND
Medical Bondage: Race, Gender, and the Origins of American Gynecology
   by Dierdre Cooper Owens

Period Repair Manual: Natural Treatment for Better Hormones and Better Periods by Lara Briden, ND

Unwell Women: Misdiagnosis and Myth in A Man-Made World by Elinor Cleghorn

The XX Brain: The Groundbreaking Science Empowering Women to Maximize Cognitive Health and Prevent Alzheimer's Disease by Lisa Mosconi, PhD

EMOTIONAL HEALTH

Anchored: How to Befriend Your Nervous System Using Polyvagal Theory by Deb Dana

It's OK That You're Not OK: Meeting Grief and Loss in a Culture That Doesn't Understand by Megan Devine

Managing Transitions (25th Anniversary Edition): Making the Most of Change by William Bridges and Susan Bridges

Radical Compassion: Learning to Love Yourself and Your World with the Practice of Rain by Tara Brach

Self-Compassion: The Proven Power of Being Kind to Yourself by Kristin Neff

OTHER

The Body Is Not an Apology: The Power of Radical Self-Love by Sonya Renee Taylor

Invisible Women: Data Bias in a World Designed for Men by Caroline Criado Perez

This Chair Rocks: A Manifesto against Ageism by Ashton Applewhite

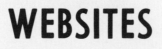

WEBSITES

Health at Every Size Health Sheets (haeshealthsheets.com)

Hot Flash Inc. (hotflashinc.com)

The North American Menopause Society (www.menopause.org)

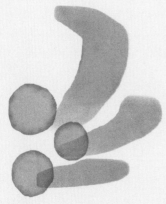

REFERENCES

CHAPTER 1: THE BASICS: AN OVERVIEW OF YOUR BODY, REPRODUCTIVE LIFE CYCLE, AND MENOPAUSAL TRANSITION

American College of Obstetricians and Gynecologists Committee Opinion No. 651. "Menstruation in Girls and Adolescents: Using the Menstrual Cycle as a Vital Sign." *Obstetrics and Gynecology* 126, no. 6 (December 2015): e143–e146. https://doi.org/10.1097/AOG.0000000000001215.

Briden, Lara, ND. *Hormone Repair Manual: Every Woman's Guide to Healthy Hormones after 40.* GreenPeak Publishing, 2021: 36.

Center for Disease Control and Prevention. "COVID-19 Racial and Ethnic Health Disparities." https://www.cdc.gov/coronavirus/2019-ncov/community/health-equity/racial-ethnic-disparities/disparities-deaths.html.

Dillaway, Heather, Mary Byrnes, Sara Miller, and Sonica Rehan. "Talking 'Among Us': How Women from Different Racial-Ethnic Groups Define and Discuss Menopause." *Health Care for Women International* 29, no. 7 (2008): 766–81. https://doi.org/10.1080/07399330802179247.

Ee, Carolyn. "A Shift in Social Attitudes Can Make Menopause a More Positive Experience." The Conversation, February 10, 2016. https://theconversation.com/a-shift-in-social-attitudes-can-make-menopause-a-positive-experience-46742.

Garbes, Angela. "What I Gained from Having a Miscarriage: When It Comes to Pregnancy Loss, There's So Much We Don't Talk About or Understand." *The Stranger*, April 27, 2016.

Gunter, Jen. "What Is Considered 'Early' for Menopause?" *New York Times*, March 7, 2019.

Harlow, S.D., S.-A.M. Burnett-Bowie, G.A. Greendale, et al. "Disparities in Reproductive Aging and Midlife Health between Black and White Women: The Study of Women's Health across the Nation (SWAN)." *Women's Midlife Health* 8, no. 3 (2022). https://doi.org/10.1186/s40695-022-00073-y.

Harlow, S.D., C. Karvonen-Gutierrez, M.R. Elliott, et al. "It Is Not Just Menopause: Symptom Clustering in the Study of Women's Health across the Nation." *Women's Midlife Health* 3, no. 2 (2017). https://doi.org/10.1186/s40695-017-0021-y.

Hasudungan, Armando. "Endocrinology—Overview." Video. YouTube, October 1, 2013. https://www.youtube.com/watch?v=YcPicFL5Jnw.

———. "Female Reproductive System—Menstrual Cycle Hormones and Regulation." Video. YouTube, July 28, 2014. https://www.youtube.com/watch?v=2_0wp8kNMus.

Hendren, Sara. *What Can a Body Do? How We Meet the Built World*. Riverhead Books, 2020: 11.

Hendrickson-Jack, Lisa. *The Fifth Vital Sign: Master Your Cycles and Optimize Your Fertility*. Fertility Friday, 2019: 96–7.

Laundau, Elizabeth. "How Much Did Grandmothers Influence Human Evolution?" *Smithsonian Magazine*, January 4, 2021.

Mattern, Susan P. *The Slow Moon Climbs: The Science, History, and Meaning of Menopause*. Princeton University Press, 2021.

Melby, M.K., M. Lock, and P. Kaufert. "Culture and Symptom Reporting at Menopause." *Human Reproduction Update* 11, no. 5 (September/October 2005): 495–512. https://doi.org/10.1093/humupd/dmi018.

Moscone, Lisa. "How Menopause Affects the Brain." Filmed December 2019 at TEDWomen. Video, 12:55. https://www.ted.com/talks/lisa_mosconi_how_menopause_affects_the_brain.

North American Menopause Society. *Menopause Practice: A Clinician's Guide*. 6th ed. North American Menopause Society, 2019.

Pagán, Angélica Marie, Vanessa Quintana, and Jenine Spotnitz. "Mitigating Black Maternal Mortality." *Berkeley Public Policy Journal* (Spring 2020). https://bppj.berkeley.edu/2020/04/13/spring -2020-journal-mitigating-black-maternal-mortality/.

Paradies, Y., J. Ben, N. Denson, et al. "Racism As a Determinant of Health: A Systematic Review and Meta-Analysis." *PLOS One* 10 no. 9 (September 23, 2015): e0138511. https://doi.org/10.1371 /journal.pone.0138511.

Peacock, K., and K.M. Ketvertis. "Menopause." *StatPearls* [Internet] (January 2022; updated February 2, 2022). https://www.ncbi.nlm.nih.gov/books/NBK507826/.

Planned Parenthood. "What's Intersex?" https://www.plannedparenthood.org/learn/gender-identity /sex-gender-identity/whats-intersex.

Singh, G.K., G.P. Daus, M. Allender, et al. "Social Determinants of Health in the United States: Addressing Major Health Inequality Trends for the Nation, 1935–2016." *International Journal of Maternal and Child Health and AIDS* 6, no. 2 (2017): 139–64. https://doi.org/10.21106/ijma.236.

Speroff, Leon, and Marc A. Fritz. *Clinical Gynecologic Endocrinology and Infertility*. 9th ed. Lippincott Williams and Wilkins, 2019.

Spitzer, Denise. "More Than the Change: Diversity and Flexibility in Menopausal Experience." In *Hot Flashes: Women Writers on the Change of Life*, edited by Lynne Taetzsch, 115–31. Faber and Faber, 1995.

Steinke, Darcey. *Flash Count Diary: Menopause and the Vindication of Natural Life*. Picador, 2020.

Swanson-Kauffman, Kristen M. "The Unborn One: A Profile of the Human Experience of Miscarriage." PhD diss., University of Colorado School of Nursing, 1983.

Taylor, Sonya Renee. *The Body Is Not an Apology: The Power of Radical Self-Love*. Berrett-Koehler Publishers, 2018: 29.

CHAPTER 2: IT'S (NOT JUST) ABOUT YOUR BODY

Applewhite, Ashton. *This Chair Rocks: A Manifesto against Ageism.* Celadon Books, 2019: 98, 117, 125, 209.

Beck, Koa. *White Feminism: From Suffragettes to Influencers, and Who They Leave Behind.* Atria Books, 2021.

Cleghorn, Elinor. *Unwell Women: Misdiagnosis and Myth in a Man-Made World.* Dutton, 2021.

Cooper Owens, Deirdre. *Medical Bondage: Race, Gender, and the Origins of American Gynecology.* The University of Georgia Press, 2017.

Corrina, Heather. *What Fresh Hell Is This?: Perimenopause, Menopause, Other Indignities, and You.* Hachette Books, 2021.

Criado Perez, Caroline. *Invisible Women: Data Bias in a World Designed for Men.* Harry N. Abrams, 2021.

Czerwiec, M.K., Ian Williams, Susan Merrill Squier, Michael J. Green, Kimberly R. Myers, and Scott T. Smith. *Graphic Medicine Manifesto.* 1st ed. Penn State University Press, 2015.

Davis, Lisa Selin. "The $10 billion Business of Perimenopause." *Fast Company*, April 19, 2021.

———. "Why Modern Medicine Keeps Overlooking Menopause." *New York Times*, April 6, 2021.

Dillaway, Heather. "Living in Uncertain Times: Experiences of Menopause and Reproductive Aging." In *The Palgrave Handbook of Critical Menstruation Studies*, edited by C. Bobel, I.T. Winkler, B. Fahs, K.A. Hasson, E.A. Kissling, and T.A. Roberts, 253–68. Palgrave Macmillan, Singapore, 2020. https://doi.org/10.1007/978-981-15-0614-7_21.

Dillaway, Heather, and Jean Burton. "'Not Done Yet?!' Women Discuss the 'End' of Menopause." *Women's Studies* 40 (2011): 149–76. https://doi.org/10.1080/00497878.2011.537982.

Dillaway, Heather, Mary Byrnes, Sara Miller, and Sonica Rehan. "Talking 'Among Us': How Women from Different Racial-Ethnic Groups Define and Discuss Menopause." *Health Care for Women*

International 29, no. 7 (2008): 766–81.
https://doi.org/10.1080/07399330802179247.

Ehrenreich, Barbara. *Witches, Midwives, and Nurses: A History of Women Healers*. 2nd ed. Feminist Press at CUNY, 2010.

Glyde, Tania. "Queer Menopause: Where Gender, Sexuality, and Age Collide." Filmed March 29, 2020. Video, 43:08.
https://www.youtube.com/watch?v=7g8eb20jBZ4.

Goldman, Leslie. "For Women of Color, Menopause Is Different," Oprah Daily, April 18, 2022. https://www.oprahdaily.com/life/health/a39649768/women-of-color-menopause/.

Hamad, Ruby. *White Tears, Brown Scars: How White Feminism Betrays Women of Color*. Catapult, 2020.

Harlow, S.D., S.-A.M. Burnett-Bowie, G.A. Greendale, et al. "Disparities in Reproductive Aging and Midlife Health between Black and White Women: The Study of Women's Health across the Nation (SWAN)." *Women's Midlife Health* 8, no. 3 (2022).
https://doi.org/10.1186/s40695-022-00073-y.

Houck, Judith A. *Hot and Bothered: Women, Medicine, and Menopause in Modern America*. 1st ed. Harvard University Press, 2008: 12–13.

Laing, Olivia. *Every Body: A Book about Freedom*. W.W. Norton, 2021.

Lennon, Kathleen. "Feminist Perspectives on the Body." The Stanford Encyclopedia of Philosophy (website). Fall 2019 ed. Edited by Edward N. Zalta. https://plato.stanford.edu/archives/fall2019/entries/feminist-body/.

Lenz, Lyz. *Belabored: A Vindication of the Rights of Pregnant Women*. Bold Type Books, 2020: 94.

Levine, Beth. "What Experts Want Women of Color to Know about Menopause." Everyday Health, January 13, 2022.
https://www.everydayhealth.com/menopause/what-experts-want-bipoc-women-to-know-about-menopause/.

Mattern, Susan P. *The Slow Moon Climbs: The Science, History, and Meaning of Menopause*. Princeton University Press, 2021.

McQueen, Ann Marie. "Mona Eltahawy Could Hot Flash to the Moon." December 3, 2021. The Hotflash Inc Podcast. https://podcasts.bcast.fm/trailer-welcome-to-the-hotflash-inc-podcast.

McVean, Ada, BSc. "The History of Hysteria." McGill Office for Science and Society, July 2017. https://www.mcgill.ca/oss/article/history-quackery/history-hysteria.

Silliman, Jael, Marlene Gerber Fried, Loretta Ross, and Elena Gutiérrez. *Undivided Rights: Women of Color Organizing for Reproductive Justice*. Haymarket Books, 2016.

Tasca, C., M. Rapetti, M.G. Carta, and B. Fadda. "Women and Hysteria in the History of Mental Health." *Clinical Practice and Epidemiology in Mental Health* 8 (2012): 110–19. https://doi.org/10.217 4/1745017901208010110.

Taylor, Sonya Renee. *The Body Is Not an Apology: The Power of Radical Self-Love*. Berrett-Koehler, 2018.

Tolentino, Jia. *Trick Mirror: Reflections on Self-Delusion*. Random House, 2020: 93.

Wolff, Jennifer. "What Doctors Don't Know about Menopause." *AARP The Magazine* (August/September 2018).

CHAPTER 3: ALL THAT COULD HAPPEN FROM PERI- TO POSTMENOPAUSE

American College of Obstetricians and Gynecologists. "Heavy Menstrual Bleeding FAQs." Updated May 2021. https://www.acog.org/womens-health/faqs/heavy-menstrual-bleeding.

Applewhite, Ashton. *This Chair Rocks: A Manifesto against Ageism*. Celadon Books, 2019.

Block, Jennifer. *Everything below the Waist: Why Healthcare Needs a Feminist Revolution*. St. Martin's Press, 2019.

Bluming, Avril, MD, and Carol Tavris, PhD. *Estrogen Matters: Why Taking Hormones in Menopause Can Improve Women's Well-Being and*

Lengthen Their Lives—Without Raising the Risk of Breast Cancer. Little, Brown Spark, 2018.

Breus, Michael J., PhD. "Menopause and Your Sleep Cycle: This Major Shift Can Bring Significant Challenges to Sleep," *Psychology Today*, June 28, 2018. https://www.psychologytoday.com/us/blog /sleep-newzzz/201806/menopause-and-your-sleep-cycle.

Briden, Lara, ND. *Hormone Repair Manual: Every Woman's Guide to Healthy Hormones after 40*. GreenPeak Publishing, 2021.

Carpenter, Laura, and John DeLamater. *Sex for Life: From Virginity to Viagra, How Sexuality Changes throughout Our Lives*. NYU Press, 2012.

Cleveland Clinic Health Library. "Estrogen and Hormones." Updated April 29, 2019. https://my.clevelandclinic.org/health /articles/16979-estrogen--hormones.

Corinna, Heather. *What Fresh Hell Is This?: Perimenopause, Menopause, Other Indignities, and You*. Hachette Books, 2021.

Devine, Megan. *It's OK That You're Not OK: Meeting Grief and Loss in a Culture That Doesn't Understand*. 1st ed. Sounds True, 2017: 17–19.

Dillaway, H. "Living in Uncertain Times: Experiences of Menopause and Reproductive Aging." In *The Palgrave Handbook of Critical Menstruation Studies*, edited by C. Bobel, I.T. Winkler, B. Fahs, K.A. Hasson, E.A. Kissling, and T.A. Roberts, 253–68. Palgrave Macmillan, Singapore, 2020. https://doi.org/10.1007/978-981 -15-0614-7_21.

Greendale, G.A., C.A. Derby, and P.M. Maki. "Perimenopause and Cognition." *Obstetrics and Gynecology Clinics of North America* 38, no. 3 (2011): 519–35. https://doi.org/10.1016/j.ogc.2011.05.007.

Gunter, Jen, MD. *The Menopause Manifesto: Own Your Health with Facts and Feminism*. Citadel, 2021.

Harvard Health Publishing. "Gender Matters: Heart Disease Risk in Women." March 25, 2017. https://www.health.harvard.edu/heart -health/gender-matters-heart-disease-risk-in-women.

———. "Hot Flashes and Heart Health: This Symptom Is Common in Menopause, but Frequent or Persistent Episodes Could Be a Sign of a Higher Risk for Heart Attack or Stroke." January 1, 2020. https://www.health.harvard.edu/womens-health/hot-flashes -and-heart-health.

Khosla, Sundeep, MD, Merry Jo Oursler, PhD, and David G. Monroe, PhD. "Estrogen and the Skeleton." *Trends in Endocrinology and Metabolism* 213, no. 11 (November 2012). https://www.ncbi.nlm.nih.gov/pmc/articles/PMC3424385/.

Lennon, Kathleen. "Feminist Perspectives on the Body." The Stanford Encyclopedia of Philosophy (website). Fall 2019 ed. Edited by Edward N. Zalta. https://plato.stanford.edu/archives/fall2019/entries/feminist-body/.

Marturana Winderl, Amy, CPT. "This Is Exactly What Happens to Your Body When You Eat a Ton of Sugar." *Self*, December 2015.

Mosconi, Lisa, PhD. *The XX Brain: The Groundbreaking Science Empowering Women to Maximize Cognitive Health and Prevent Alzheimer's Disease*. Illustrated ed. Avery, 2020.

Nagoski, Emily. *Come As You Are: The Surprising New Science That Will Transform Your Sex Life*. Updated ed. Simon and Schuster, 2021.

North American Menopause Society. "Can Menopause Be Blamed for Increased Forgetfulness and Lack of Attention?" January 13, 2021. https://www.menopause.org/docs/default-source/press-release/cognitive-changes-during-the-menopausal-transition-1-13-21.pdf.

———. *Menopause Practice: A Clinician's Guide*. 6th ed. North American Menopause Society, 2019.

Roman-Blas, Jorge A., Santos Castaneda, Raquel Largo, and Gabriel Herrero-Beaumont. "Osteoarthritis Associated with Estrogen Deficiency." *Arthritis Research and Therapy* (September 2009). https://www.ncbi.nlm.nih.gov/pmc/articles/PMC2787275/.

Sheehy, Gail. *The Silent Passage: Menopause*. Random House New York, 1992: 40.

Sole-Smith, Virginia. *The Eating Instinct: Food Culture, Body Image, and Guilt in America*. Henry Holt, 2018.

———. "What If Doctors Stopped Prescribing Weight Loss?" *Scientific American*, July 1, 2020.

Speroff, Leon, and Marc A. Fritz. *Clinical Gynecologic Endocrinology and Infertility*. 9th ed. Lippincott Williams and Wilkins, 2019.

Strings, Sabrina, and Lindo Bacon. "The Racist Roots of Fighting Obesity." *Scientific American*, June 4, 2020.

Winterich, Julie A. "Sex, Menopause, and Culture: Sexual Orientation
and the Meaning of Menopause for Women's Sex Lives." *Gender
and Society* 17, no. 4 (2003): 627–42.
https://doi.org/10.1177/0891243203253962.
You Magazine. "How Gynaecologist Dr. Jennifer Gunter Handles
the Menopause." May 16, 2021. https://www.you.co.uk
/how-gynaecologist-dr-jennifer-gunter-handles-the-menopause/.

CHAPTER 4: CHANGE IN YOUR BODY CHANGES YOU

Bridges, William, and Susan Bridges. *Managing Transitions: Making
the Most of Change*. Special 25th anniversary ed. Da Capo Lifelong
Books, 2017.
Calhoun, Ada. "The New Midlife Crisis." Oprah.com, October 5, 2017.
https://www.oprah.com/sp/new-midlife-crisis.html.
Devine, Megan. *It's OK That You're Not OK: Meeting Grief and Loss in
a Culture That Doesn't Understand*. 1st ed. Sounds True, 2017: 34,
45–9, 57–61.
———. "Stitching Opportunity into Crisis Can Erase Pain That
Needs to Be Felt." Interview by Kimberly Adams. *Marketplace*,
NPR, December 29, 2020. Audio, 5:47. https://www.marketplace
.org/2020/12/29/how-grief-manifests-economy/.
Dillaway, Heather E. "(Un)Changing Menopausal Bodies: How
Women Think and Act in the Face of a Reproductive Transition and
Gendered Beauty Ideals." *Sex Roles* 53, no. 1–2 (2005): 1–17.
https://doi.org/10.1007/S11199-005-4269-6.
May, Katherine. *Wintering: The Power of Rest and Retreat in Difficult
Times*. 1st ed. Riverhead Books, 2020.
Schwedel, Heather. "Marina Benjamin on What We Don't Talk about
When We Talk about Women and Aging." Slate, March 28, 2017.
https://slate.com/human-interest/2017/03/talking-about

-women-aging-and-menopause-with-marina-benjamin-author
-of-the-middlepause.html.

Solnit, Rebecca. *The Mother of All Questions*. Later printing ed.
Haymarket Books, 2017: 5–6.

CHAPTER 5:
GETTING READY

Oster, Emily. "Get Your Family Running More Smoothly with
Tricks from Running Small Businesses." Interview by Elise Hu.
Life Kit, NPR, August 9, 2021. Audio, 17:00.
https://www.npr.org/2021/08/06/1025447008/emily-oster-the
-family-firm-decision-making-parenting.

CHAPTER 6:
GETTING RELIEF

American Pharmacists Association. "Frequently Asked Questions
about Pharmaceutical Compounding." https://pharmacist.com
/Practice/Patient-Care-Services/Compounding
/Compounding-FAQs.

André, Christophe. "Proper Breathing Brings Better Health." *Scientific
American*, January 15, 2019. https://www.scientificamerican.com
/article/proper-breathing-brings-better-health/.

Barrett, Lisa Felman, PhD. "Try These Two Smart Techniques to Help
You Master Your Emotions." Ideas.TED.com, June 21, 2018.
https://ideas.ted.com/try-these-two-smart-techniques-to-help
-you-master-your-emotions/.

Cagnacci, A., S. Arangino, A. Renzi, A.L. Zanni, S. Malmusi, and
A. Volpe. "Kava-Kava Administration Reduces Anxiety in

Perimenopausal Women." *Maturitas* 44, no. 2 (February 25, 2003):103–9. https://doi.org/10.1016/s0378-5122(02)00317-1. PMID: 12590005.

Centers for Disease Control and Prevention. "Benefits of Physical Activity." April 5, 2021. https://www.cdc.gov/physicalactivity /basics/pa-health/index.htm.

———. "Dietary Guidelines for Alcohol." April 19, 2022. https://www.cdc.gov/alcohol/fact-sheets/moderate-drinking.htm.

Chatterjee, Rhitu. "Sitting Too Much Drags Down Your Mental Health. Here's How to Get Moving." NPR, October 16, 2021. https://www .npr.org/sections/health-shots/2021/10/16/1034201715/home -workout-exercise-tips.

Choi, Y.J., S.K. Myung, and J.H. Lee. "Light Alcohol Drinking and Risk of Cancer: A Meta-Analysis of Cohort Studies." *Cancer Research and Treatment* 50, no. 2 (April 2018): 474–87. https://doi.org/10.4143 /crt.2017.094. PMID: 28546524; PMCID: PMC5912140.

Cleghorn, Elinor. *Unwell Women: Misdiagnosis and Myth in a Man-Made World*. Dutton, 2021.

Eatemadnia, A., S. Ansari, P. Abedi, and S. Najar. "The Effect of *Hypericum perforatum* on Postmenopausal Symptoms and Depression: A Randomized Controlled Trial." *Complementary Therapies in Medicine* 45 (August 2019): 109–13. https://doi .org/10.1016/j.ctim.2019.05.028. PMID: 31331546.

Faubion, S.S., R. Sood, J.M. Thielen, and L.T. Shuster. "Caffeine and menopausal symptoms: what is the association?" *Menopause* 22, no. 2 (February 2015): 155–58. https://doi.org/10.1097 /GME.0000000000000301. PMID: 25051286.

Felton, Ryan. "The FDA's Tattered Safety Net for Dietary Supplements." *Consumer Reports*, October 15, 2020. https://www.consumerreports.org/dietary-supplements /fdas-supplement-warning-system-has-deadly-limitations/.

Fields, Jay. "An Uncommon Fill-Up, and Other Words That Start with F." Blog. http://jay-fields.com/writings/2019/8/20/an-uncommon -fill-up-and-other-words-that-start-with-f.

Food and Drug Administration. "Compounding and the FDA: Questions and Answers." https://www.fda.gov/drugs/human

-drug-compounding/compounding-and-fda-questions
-and-answers.

Fournier, A., S. Mesrine, L. Dossus, M.C. Boutron-Ruault, F. Clavel-Chapelon, and N. Chabbert-Buffet. "Risk of Breast Cancer after Stopping Menopausal Hormone Therapy in the E3N Cohort." *Breast Cancer Research and Treatment* 145, no. 2 (June 2014): 535–43. https://doi.org/10.1007/s10549-014-2934-6. Erratum in *Breast Cancer Research and Treatment* 147, no. 1 (August 2014): 225. PMID: 24781971; PMCID: PMC5924370.

Grant, Adam. "There's a Name for the Blah You're Feeling: It's Called Languishing." *New York Times*, April 19, 2021. https://www.nytimes.com/2021/04/19/well/mind/covid-mental-health-languishing.html.

Gunter, Jen, MD. *The Menopause Manifesto: Own Your Health with Facts and Feminism*. Citadel, 2021.

Haspel, Tamar. "Most Dietary Supplements Don't Do Anything. Why Do We Spend $35 Billion a Year on Them?" *Washington Post*, January 27, 2020. https://www.washingtonpost.com/lifestyle/food/most-dietary-supplements-dont-do-anything-why-do-we-spend-35-billion-a-year-on-them/2020/01/24/947d2970-3d62-11ea-baca-eb7ace0a3455_story.html.

Houck, Judith A. *Hot and Bothered: Women, Medicine, and Menopause in Modern America*. Harvard University Press, 2006.

Hudson, Tori, ND. "Ashwagandha for Improving Sleep Quality." Blog, April 26, 2021. https://drtorihudson.com/general/ashwagandha-for-improving-sleep-quality/.

———. "Maca for Anti-Depressant Induced Sexual Dysfunction." Blog, October 30, 2015. https://drtorihudson.com/general/maca-for-anti-depressant-induced-sexual-dysfunction/.

———. "Theanine for Anxiety . . . I'm Sure Many of Us Could Use It!" Blog, March 11, 2022. https://drtorihudson.com/general/theanine-for-anxiety-im-sure-many-of-us-could-use-it/.

Kazemi, F., S.Z. Masoumi, A. Shayan, and K. Oshvandi. "The Effect of Evening Primrose Oil Capsule on Hot Flashes and Night Sweats in Postmenopausal Women: A Single-Blind Randomized Controlled Trial." *Journal of Menopausal Medicine* 27, no. 1 (April 2021): 8–14.

https://doi.org/10.6118/jmm.20033. PMID: 33942584; PMCID: PMC8102809.

Lamott, Anne. "Anne Lamott: Radical Self-Care Changes Everything." Interview by Tami Simon. Sounds True: Insights at the Edge podcast, November 23, 2021. Audio 54:00. https://podcasts.apple .com/us/podcast/anne-lamott-radical-self-care-changes -everything/id307934313?i=1000392723918.

Loria, Kevin. "How to Choose Supplements Wisely." *Consumer Reports,* October 30, 2019. https://www.consumerreports.org /supplements/how-to-choose-supplements-wisely-a2238386100/.

Mattern, Susan P. *The Slow Moon Climbs: The Science, History, and Meaning of Menopause.* Princeton University Press, 2021.

Mosconi, Lisa, PhD. *The XX Brain: The Groundbreaking Science Empowering Women to Maximize Cognitive Health and Prevent Alzheimer's Disease.* Illustrated ed. Avery, 2020.

National Institutes of Health (NIH). "Relaxation Techniques: What You Need To Know." June 2021. https://www.nccih.nih.gov/health /relaxation-techniques-what-you-need-to-know.

NIH, Office of Dietary Supplements. "What You Need to Know: Dietary Supplements." Updated September 3, 2020. https://ods.od.nih.gov/factsheets/WYNTK-Consumer/.

North American Menopause Society. "Effective Treatments for Sexual Problems." http://www.menopause.org/for-women /sexual-health-menopause-online/effective-treatments-for -sexual-problems.

———. *Menopause Practice: A Clinician's Guide.* 6th ed. North American Menopause Society, 2019.

Oster, Emily. "Health Recommendations and Selection in Health Behaviors." *American Economic Review: Insights* 2, no. 2 (June 2020): 143–60. https://doi.org/10.1257/aeri.20190355.

Palmisano, Brian T., Lin Zhu, and John M. Stafford. "Estrogens in the Regulation of Liver Lipid Metabolism." *Advances in Experimental Medicine and Biology* 1043 (2017): 227–56. https://www.ncbi.nlm .nih.gov/pmc/articles/PMC5763482/.

Pittler, Max H., MD, and Edzard Ernst, MD, PhD, FRCPC (Edin). "Efficacy of Kava Extract for Treating Anxiety: Systematic Review and Meta-Analysis." *Journal of Clinical Psychopharmacology* 20, no. 1 (February 2000): 84–89.

Pkhaladze, L., N. Davidova, A. Khomasuridze, R. Shengelia, and A.G. Panossian. "*Actaea racemosa* L. Is More Effective in Combination with *Rhodiola rosea* L. for Relief of Menopausal Symptoms: A Randomized, Double-Blind, Placebo-Controlled Study." *Pharmaceuticals (Basel)* 13, no. 5 (May 21, 2020): 102. https://doi.org/10.3390/ph13050102.

Rubin, Courtney. "How to Manage Your New-Year Expectations." *New York Times*, December 26, 2020. https://www.nytimes .com/2020/12/26/well/new-year-expectations.html.

Safran Foer, Jonathan. "Jonathan Safran Foer on Marriage, Religion, and Universal Balances." Interview by Terry Gross. *Fresh Air*, NPR, July 7, 2017. Audio 37:00. https://www.npr.org/2017/07/07/535969620/jonathan-safran-foer -on-marriage-religion-and-universal-balances.

Shinjyo, N., G. Waddell, and J. Green. "Valerian Root in Treating Sleep Problems and Associated Disorders—A Systematic Review and Meta-Analysis." *Journal of Evidence-Based Integrative Medicine* 25 (January/December 2020): 2515690X20967323. https://doi.org/10.1177/2515690X20967323. PMID: 33086877; PMCID: PMC7585905.

Stefanick, Marcia L., PhD. "Estrogens and Progestins: Background and History, Trends in Use, and Guidelines and Regimens Approved by the U.S. Food and Drug Administration." *The American Journal of Medicine* 118, no. 12B (2005): 64S–73S. https://www.amjmed.com /article/S0002-9343(05)00919-8/pdf.

Sternfeld, Barbara, and Sheila Dugan. "Physical Activity and Health During the Menopausal Transition." *Obstetrics and Gynecology Clinics of North America* 38, no. 3 (2011): 537–66. https://doi.org/10.1016/j.ogc.2011.05.008.

CHAPTER 7:
GETTING SUPPORT

Ahmed, Sara. *Living a Feminist Life*. Illustrated ed. Duke University Press, 2017.

Beck, Koa. *White Feminism: From Suffragettes to Influencers, and Who They Leave Behind*. Atria Books, 2021.

Boss, Pauline. "Navigating Loss without Closure." Interview by Krista Tippett. On Being podcast, June 23, 2016. Audio, 51:00. https://onbeing.org/programs/pauline-boss-navigating-loss-without-closure/.

Devine, Megan. *It's OK That You're Not OK: Meeting Grief and Loss in a Culture That Doesn't Understand*. 1st ed. Sounds True, 2017.

North American Menopause Society. "What's an NCMP?" https://www.menopause.org/for-women/whats-an-ncmp.

Vedantam, Shankar. "A Social Prescription: Why Human Connection Is Crucial to Our Health." *Hidden Brain*, NPR, April 20, 2020. Audio, 49:00. https://www.npr.org/2020/04/20/838757183/a-social-prescription-why-human-connection-is-crucial-to-our-health.

Zoltan, Vanessa, and Casper ter Kuile. "Are You Okay?" The Real Question podcast, August 9, 2021. Audio, 43:00. https://play.acast.com/s/the-real-question/areyouokay-.

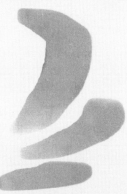

ABOUT THE AUTHORS

Sasha Davies is a writer of nonfiction. Her work focuses on making topics that are traditionally the purview of experts more accessible and inviting to a broader audience. Her previous books include *The Guide to West Coast Cheese: More than 300 Cheeses Handcrafted in California, Oregon, and Washington*, and *The Cheesemaker's Apprentice: An Insider's Guide to the Art and Craft of Homemade Artisan Cheese, Taught by the Masters*.

She lives in the Pacific Northwest and is an avid lover of the outdoors.

Tori Hudson, ND, is a naturopathic physician and clinical professor at the National University of Naturopathic Medicine, Southwest College of Naturopathic Medicine, Canadian College of Naturopathic Medicine, and Bastyr University. Dr. Hudson has been in practice for more than thirty-eight years; is the medical director of her clinic, A Woman's Time, in Portland, Oregon; and is also the founder and codirector of Naturopathic Education and Residency Consortium, a nonprofit organization for accredited naturopathic residencies. She is a nationally recognized expert on menopause and author of the *Women's Encyclopedia of Natural Medicine*.